Health

Recklessly Abandoned

Health Recklessly Abandoned

Take Back Control of Your Own Health and Live the Life You Deserve

Dr. Vincent Bellonzi

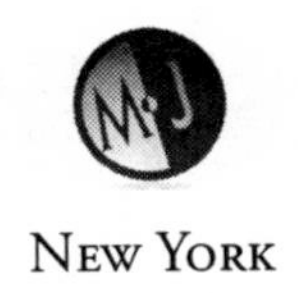

New York

Health Recklessly Abandoned

Take Back Control of Your Own Health and Live the Life You Deserve

ISBN 978-1-61448-431-8 paperback
ISBN 978-1-61448-432-5 eBook
Library of Congress Control Number: 2012950212

Morgan James Publishing
The Entrepreneurial Publisher
5 Penn Plaza, 23rd Floor,
New York City, New York 10001
(212) 655-5470 office • (516) 908-4496 fax
www.MorganJamesPublishing.com

Cover Design by:
Rachel Lopez
www.r2cdesign.com

Interior Design by:
Bonnie Bushman
bonnie@caboodlegraphics.com

Table of Contents

Introduction

Have You Recklessly Abandoned Your Health?

There is a story told about a town located at the bottom of a sheer cliff. At the top of the cliff, there was a road leading right up to the edge, and a blind turn just before the edge. Very frequently, someone came down that road too quickly and went careening over the cliff. As a result of the services that it was required to provide when people went over the cliff, the town had grown appreciably. It had equipped itself with rescue personnel, ambulances, trauma centers, doctors, and a huge hospital. In fact, this town had a great reputation for saving people; they were heroes. But one had to ask, "Wouldn't it be better to find a way to keep people from careening off the cliff in the first place?"

This town's approach can serve as a metaphor not only for our current medical model, but our own approach to health. We drive too fast and recklessly sail off the cliff, grateful that the town below is so well equipped to respond to our emergency. But how much better would it have been to have anticipated the curve and stayed on the road—and not experience the emergency at all?

To get careless or reckless with something as important as your health is always a mistake. The American public at large has become negligent toward maintaining their health. In fact, they have "recklessly abandoned" their own potential for wellness. The average person in America, for all their education, does not understand how much of a part they play in their own health or wellness. People don't focus on their health until it's gone. Most people only see a health practitioner once they have developed a problem.

In conventional medicine, "prevention" revolves around the early detection of problems already in place. This requires expensive diagnostic equipment and tests, medical specialists, and then treatment of whatever is detected. But this is not prevention; this is a life rescue. The lifeguard on duty in the tower is looking for someone already in trouble. When they see someone struggling, there is a call to action, and everybody rushes to the aid of the person in distress. It is quite a spectacle, and it is commendable as well. The lifeguards and health practitioners who save lives in dire situations are true heroes.

The lifeguard scenario plays out in healthcare even for those people who seem to take a more proactive approach to their health. They develop a close relationship with practitioners who keep an eye on them, schedule early detection testing, and focus on distress management. These people also tend to assume and accept that their health will decline automatically, and they will need escalating care.

But if you peruse the studies on aging, you may be interested to discover that very few things are actually caused by aging, despite the fact we tend to blame so many of our problems on the aging process. In the majority of cases, symptoms are occurring more as the result of inattention to our lifestyle. Aches and pains, allergies and autoimmune disorders, diabetes, heart disease, and even cancer are produced through mechanisms that we now understand. Each of us plays a part in how those mechanisms proceed and, more importantly, in the end result.

Time or "aging" is not a cause of disease. You don't just "catch" disease. Your body is a composite of biological systems working in conjunction with each other. Every disease requires a mechanism for its production. The human body is always doing its best to adapt to the situation. If you're not paying attention, that adaptation may end up with negative results.

Disease and symptoms are no more than dysfunctions of the mind and of the body. There is no one who has more control over these structures or functions than yourself. When you visit the doctor and are given a prescription for medication or for some medical procedure, you have already lost control of function. You are asking for someone else to reach into their toolbox in order to take control for you. The biggest breakdown that I see is when people give up control of their bodies for far too long. Being "out of control" can happen, and it is a good thing that there are people trained to take over, to keep us safe and alive.

I am a healthcare practitioner; however, I do not desire to spend all my time saving lives. I want to be the person who journeys to the top of the cliff, or perhaps way up that road that leads to the cliff, where people have another choice. I want to tell people not to go down that road because of the cliff. That way, at least those people won't have to be saved.

I am a chiropractor, a certified health and fitness instructor, a certified strength and conditioning specialist, and board certified in nutrition. I like to put all this together and refer to myself as a "wellness advisor." After all, the word "doctor" is actually translated from the Latin word for "teacher." For the past twenty years, I have worked in a clinical setting, helping people to regain their health. For the last ten years, I have been a part of the Austin Wellness Clinic. Through those years I have worked with many who had given up the chance to feel better and live healthy lives. I have seen literally thousands of people transform their own lives and regain their health, actually reversing sometimes severe mental and physical conditions. I have witnessed people who thought they would never walk again not only walk, but actually compete in athletic or recreational activities. The steps required to achieve these results are quite straightforward:

1. Stop all processed food and consume only wholesome, real food.
2. Immediately begin some form of physical activity based on current physical abilities. For some this was walking; for others, the exercise might be simply getting up or down. Even someone who is not able to get around can exercise with modification.
3. Clean up the internal environment of the body. Often we would design a cleanse.
4. Repair the gut.
5. Ensure the availability of sufficient nutrients, as well as the targeted use of nutraceuticals (nutrients used at a higher dose to affect function).

This is exactly what we will cover in this book. I work hard to be a trusted resource, and I will simply share what I have observed in practice. It has become my intention, and my passion, to help people realize their potential. I want you to realize yours. Without your health, without energy, without a properly functioning body, I believe that people are challenged in life unnecessarily. When people understand how their body works, and the mechanisms that create disease, they are empowered.

The strategy that I am proposing creates a lifestyle plan, where we will not require the hero. Prevention would require, by definition, that the person never experience distress or, especially, the need for rescue. Prevention requires a person educated enough and trained well enough to avoid such situations. There are people who design a lifestyle that keeps their body and their mind safe and properly functioning. If they do this well enough, the issue of rescue does not arise because the fire never started. In this book, I hope to show you that your body does not make mistakes and is only responding to the way that you live your life.

Wellness is defined as a state of optimal physical, mental, and social well-being, not merely the absence of disease or infirmity. To create and to maintain a state of wellness, one is required to design and implement a lifestyle that is congruent with his or her biological systems, genomics, and ancestral evolution. I want you to know about processes you may never have heard of, like epigenitics, kinase communication, the triage that your body is forced into, and the burden created for the body when it accumulates too many toxic substances.

Symptoms do not occur out of the blue. They occur from dysfunction. There is a broken mechanism leading to or producing that symptom. The answer, ultimately, is to correct the mechanism. This is not accomplished by simply taking a pill or undergoing some procedure. It is not accomplished by medical management. Fixing broken systems depends on the total lifestyle that you live. By lifestyle, I simply mean eating proper, nutritive foods and doing challenging but not overwhelming physical activity. Improving mechanisms comes from an improved environmental exposure.

Please don't misunderstand: I am not saying that eating an apple a day will cure everything. What I am saying is that the better lifestyle design you create, the more impact you will have on improving and even resolving physical and mental problems. In life, nothing is static. If your intention is to maintain your health and vitality, then you will have to understand adaptation and know how to create it. If you don't participate in the creation of wellness, your only alternative is a maladaptive state, and your body will have a tendency to degenerate. (I will expand on these concepts throughout the rest of this book.)

Most of you reading this are well aware of the fact that you will benefit from consuming a better diet, and I'm sure that you know some of the benefits of exercise. But in this book, I do not intend to preach to you or to tell you what to do. I want to present to you reliable facts, and then I want you to make your own decisions. I want to share information I have learned and tell you about miracles I have experienced myself. I want to explore with you how with some small changes, you can see great benefit. It is not about what is right or wrong, or good or bad, but about developing a plan that produces the best results. It is about your freedom to enjoy life.

I remember playing high school football back in the day, complete with the clichéd locker room speech. I remember it like it was yesterday. We had a very, let us say, "expressive" head coach who had the capacity to be both intimidating and yet very motivating. One of his favorite expressions was the term "reckless abandon." It was our mission to play every season, every game, every play, and every minute of the game with what he called "reckless abandon." The coach wanted us to focus every bit of our brain, use all the potential of our bodies, and tap into every bit of our being. He wanted us to invest everything that we had in the game. The coach wanted us "all in" and not to hold anything back. He wanted us to leave the field with no regrets because we had given it our best effort.

I understand now that what the coach wanted was for us to be fully present and to push ourselves to excel. He wanted us to ask ourselves for that 120 percent effort and go beyond our preconceived limits. He wanted us to demonstrate to ourselves the true potential that we all possess. My high school coach understood that people have a tendency to hold back and play it safe. When something important is on the line, the winners reach beyond safety and come up with the victory.

There are certain times in our lives when every one of us will need to reach beyond what we believe we can accomplish and actually excel beyond our expectations. We all need to approach our priorities with the intensity of reckless abandon, so that rationalization does not detour us from our goals.

Are you ready to pursue your health with reckless abandon? I want you to be motivated, and I want you to win when something important is on the line. I believe in all of you, just like the coach believed in us. I see potential in all of my patients, and I am confident that anyone reading this book can have a winning future. Most important of all, I know that you can improve on and maximize a state of optimal health for yourself.

I have seen too many people who have abandoned their own physical health and vitality. Of course, it happened slowly; as the years pass people get busy with life, while physical fitness and wellness are given very low priority. These are the people who come to our clinic with fatigue, brain fog, pain, and many other physical dysfunctions. It does not have to be that way. These people have been reckless with their health, and I want every one of them, including you, to get it back.

But this book isn't just for those who have decided to abandon their health themselves, one decision at a time. I have also worked with paraplegics and even a quadriplegic. I was amazed at what they could accomplish if they just went for it. I have worked with thousands of people who had accommodated to their condition, whatever the cause. Allergies, joint pains, gastrointestinal dysfunctions, fatigue, sleep disruption, hormonal imbalance, and the list goes on. These patients were amazed when symptoms simply vanished as function was restored. Not by using medication, not by magic, but by doing no more than understanding how the body works, and working with it.

I hear every day from people who are told they will never be free from medical management. What I want to explain to you is that freedom is not free; it requires effort, and even some sacrifice. But the freedom provided by health is real. Anyone can become stronger and healthier than they are today. So many of us have resigned ourselves to the life of the "walking wounded" and believe that there is no choice. I hope that as you read this book you will gain an understanding of how your body works, and how to keep it working well.

This entire book is really just an introduction of concepts. It's not the end; it is a beginning—a proposal, if you'll allow that. I propose that you and I, and as many people as we can reach, learn how to create and experience healthy, vital lives. I will continue in the future to explore new science and new ideas, and I invite you to join me by visiting (www.recklesshealth.com). You don't have to recklessly abandon your health. You can pursue it with reckless abandon.

Are you in the game?

Chapter 1

Reckless Abandon

A Strategy to Create Health

We live in a "no-fault" society. Pervasive in our culture is the concept that you are entitled to all the rights but bear none of the responsibilities. This can be easily demonstrated by examining the medical-industrial complex that exists in our country and, for that matter, around the world. Prevention has come to mean finding a disease in an early stage, and then treating it. These treatments are very profitable for some big corporations and may be dogmatically viewed as necessary for the entire duration of a patient's life. Of course, I propose that treatment be initiated when it is necessary to deal with a disease process, but that in the large majority of cases, with the right strategy, treatment is short and defined. As soon as function is restored to the body, treatment ends and the road to health is resumed. "Treatment" is really a short-term solution, or a stop-gap strategy used until body function is restored. When we identify the disease pattern, then we understand better the mechanism of each disease and also have a strategy to undo it.

In the "no-fault" medical-industrial complex, you are told that you are healthy until something goes seriously wrong, and a disease can be identified and labeled (aka the diagnosis). In fact, I have seen patients who were told to wait until things were bad enough so that they could be diagnosed, or properly categorized. It is only when a patient is experiencing the fulminant disease that the patient is allowed to begin treatment with standardized protocols. Early stages and signs of dysfunction are often ignored, as well as the major tools of health, which are nutrition, exercise, and reduction of toxic environmental exposure. Some conventional practitioners go so far as to tell people that they are healthy as long as they remain under medical management, and symptoms are "controlled." Symptom control is not health, whether by medication or by green pharmacy (herbs). Optimal health is the absence of symptoms and disease; it is "optimal" function. People have been led to believe that they themselves play little or no part in the creation of disease, and that without modern medicines, human beings cannot be healthy.

There is no time like the present to actually participate in our own health. When I use the term "reckless abandon," I mean "going for it" without worry or the extreme caution that keeps us all from moving forward. When it comes to your health, you just have to do it. It is so common for us to look for convenience or immediate gratification instead of keeping a focus on our health. Thinking that you do not have time for a healthy meal, so you'll "grab" something now and eat better later. Popping a pill every time you have a headache instead of finding out what caused the headache. Being too "busy" to exercise or even move out of your chair.

Rationalizations, like the above, become the health problems that we deal with later. We all seem to put our health off until there is a better time; however, a better time never seems to present itself. When we are young, we are too busy anticipating a time when we are old enough to get a car or some other "grown-up" possession. As we get older, we put no emphasis on health because we believe ourselves to be invincible. Finally, the day comes when we "get sick," and we have to seek out a doctor for something more serious than a cut or broken bone; we have contracted a disease. The doctor, using knowledge gained in years of school, works to label our problem and then proceeds to manage the disease for us.

I hear too often statements like, "I'll exercise when I have the energy," or "I'll eat better when I have time, money, etc." I am asking you to alter your paradigm and your plan just a little. The answer lies in doing the right things now, so you don't have to have your disease managed later. We have a weight-loss program in my clinic, and step one is a supportive cleanse. We have people eat only "real," unprocessed foods and take supplemental nutrients for four weeks. To a person, everyone feels better, but the more common and startling results are when allergies, headaches, and other disease symptoms that this person may have dealt with for years seem to just vanish.

A good example for a prevention strategy is diabetes. Many doctors will not even mention blood sugar levels to a patient until they appear to be outside of the laboratory ranges. Once fasting blood sugar rises above 100, then some doctors may casually remark to the patient, "Looks like you are now pre-diabetic; let's just keep an eye this," or many times the doctor will just say, "Let's wait and see what happens." Then, when your fasting blood sugar rises over 140, or when the hemoglobin A-1c is above a certain percentage and you can be diagnosed as a diabetic, now the doctor is concerned enough and starts treatment. Waiting until disease occurs and then treating the disease is not prevention. If we look at research, there is very good evidence that as a person's fasting blood sugar rises above 84 milligrams per deciliter, they enter the risk group for diabetes. Diabetes is the loss of control of sugar concentration in the blood. If you notice early that you are losing control, you can take action at this early stage and not proceed all the way to diabetes. This is true prevention.

Reckless abandon can also mean yielding to natural impulses without consideration of consequences. But I am not talking about being careless, like a bull in a china shop. Rather I am referring to the focus, concentration, and intent of a seasoned athlete looking to score and to win. The simple secret to health is to not develop disease. Years ago, Professor Louis Claude Vincent of France coined the term *biological terrain*. He was referring to the internal environment of the human body and the theory that if you keep that environment within certain parameters, you will not develop symptoms and disease. Living a proactive lifestyle can get you as near to "bulletproof" as is possible.

Our paradigm includes our actual belief about how everything works and how things are put together. It is our understood and factual pattern or model for the universe. I want to challenge your paradigm and perhaps offer you reason to change it. Sometimes your core beliefs serve you well; however, sometimes they do not. Your own genetics under certain circumstances can help you survive, but alter the environmental conditions, and you may not make it. For example, the Pima Indians in the southwestern United States were well adapted to live in the desert. However, if given access to abundant food, these same people easily develop diabetes, obesity, and heart disease, and limit their life quality and lifespan.

Our reckless abandon requires a lifestyle that is congruent with each person's genetics. Our lifestyle consists of the food choices that we make, our physical activity level, and everything that we expose ourselves to both mentally and physically. Our habits, attitudes, moral standards, economic relationships, and personal relationships all make up a way of life. One cannot discount their lifestyle as a potent contributor to health or disease. Yet there are many people who do not even consider managing their lifestyle until it is almost too late. Some of the healthiest people that I know survived cancer because they woke up upon hearing that diagnosis.

The Strategy

For many patients, good health is considered to include management by the proper medical teams, medications, vaccines, and surgical interventions. Health really means self-sufficiency from all that. If you are utilizing medications or require medical management, then you're not healthy. It actually falls upon you to restore your health by restoring the biological systems of the body to a point of proper function. For example, if you have high blood pressure, there are many things that you can do to help your body control blood pressure on its own. Hypertension is an inflammatory situation that, when corrected, tends to resolve the high blood pressure. Correction comes as the result of a proper lifestyle. As long as you utilize medication to control the blood pressure or the inflammation, you are not healthy. You are being controlled and managed by someone else. Consider yourself on life support.

The same is true if you are utilizing cholesterol-lowering drugs. For the majority of the people on statin drugs, I have found that when more information is available, we can take a more natural approach. Many people are put on statins simply because their total cholesterol was above 200mg/dl. In functional medicine, this is not enough information, and a safer approach can also be more effective. More to come on all of this in later chapters.

This book is not at all about guilt, blame, thoughtless judgments, or hopelessness. This book is truly, one hundred percent about hope and results—the hope that springs from knowing that in matters of health, you have control of your own destiny. Your health is not all predetermined by fate, by genetics, or by getting to the best doctor. There is a new understanding of the patterns of health and well-being. Scientists are now uncovering the mechanisms of physiological communication and the adaptive responses that occur from this communication both from inside and outside the human body. We determine our own health status, which is a response to how we live our life.

Again, the human body—your body—does not make mistakes. The systems and mechanisms that make up your physiology are always working to keep up with your present demands. The state of "health" demands energy for function and proper communication between those systems. Health is not demonstrated simply by lab work inside of, or outside of, a laboratory reference range. Health is demonstrated and experienced by proper function, independent of synthesized interventions like medication. Real health requires your full attention. For example, learn everything you can about how your body works and interacts with stress. Too little stress, and the body will degenerate, simply fall apart, and stop functioning. Too much stress, and the body is overwhelmed and, with too great of a burden, cannot respond appropriately. We will talk more about stress later in this book.

If you're not careful about how you design your exercise and physical activity, you may not produce your desired results either. If your only objective is to burn calories, then you tend to lose control over where those calories come from. Most people who train with low-intensity aerobic exercise alone tend to burn primarily muscle protein for energy. Exercise takes planning and cross-training. Your physical training has to include methods that maintain muscle mass; increase aerobic capacity; train balance, coordination, and stability; and improve endurance. The results you produce determine the function of your body. If you plan your exercise to improve lean tissue, enhance biological function, and shift physiology, then you finish healthier. As a trainer, I have observed many people work very hard, sometimes hours a day in their attempts to lose weight. Their final result was to gain weight and promote disease. How you exercise determines if your adaptive results will be positive or negative.

Some of you may be thinking, "But some things just happen—like someone contracting a disease at a young age, some type of accident, or just a lack of information at the right time."

Yes, I have to agree that things out of our control will happen to all of us. There is not always an easy or immediate explanation, but there is always a mechanism in place that has affected you. So, yes, the young are affected before they can play an active part in their own health. In many people, it seems that they do accidentally contract a disease or undergo a dysfunctional process. Some people get sick, some pass on before their time, and some suffer without any apparent cause or solution. However, I want to reach out to the greater majority of you who can make a difference and not create or prolong unnecessary symptoms and suffering. I implore you to live a life congruent with how *your* body works so you can experience wellness.

In my many years of practice, I have seen so many more people who have absolutely amazed me. I learned very early in life, and then in my practice, not to place limits on anyone at any time. When you choose to believe some authority or practitioner over yourself, you can easily become lost. Doctor translates to teacher, or advisor, not the all-knowing. I have seen so many people who would not accept the limits placed on them. They became truly invested in improving their own capabilities and tested the imposed constraints, if only to see for themselves. These people had a real impact on effectively reducing their recognized disease and impairment.

These "non-acceptors" simply chose to work from their current capabilities and continue to find ways to overcome their limits. Some unbelievably were told to never do physical exercise again, yet they did not want to accept this. So they modified, trained, tested, and became functional again. Some were told that their life would be cut short by disease. Again, they did not accept this as their lot in life, and they went on to live beyond all expectations. Others I met were told that all of their symptoms were to be expected or accepted at this point in their life, or were due to ethnicity or sex. They went on to prove the judgments and assumptions to be wrong. Health and physical function are dynamic, ever-changing, and cannot be ignored. Whatever your current situation, there are strategies for improving; just take a step at a time.

So what does it take to be as healthy as possible, and why would you accept any less? Like any other success, health requires your attention to all the details. Forget about counting calories; instead start examining what you are choosing to put into your own body. As stated before, I have yet to see a person who eats only "real food" have a problem with their weight. The only scientifically proven mechanisms for longevity and health are caloric restriction and exercise. Please understand that "caloric restriction" is taking in less calories, while getting more or sufficient nutrients. This requires more planning than just eating less. Many diseases of the mind and the body have been proven to be caused by a calorie intake that was too high. We do not want to create starvation, but simply lower the calorie intake. This can be accomplished by changing what you eat. Vegetables naturally contain more nutrients and fewer calories. Processed breads and cereals contain more calories, with very low if any nutrients.

Remember the book (and then the movie) *The Perfect Storm?* Everything necessary came together at once to create a weather situation of "epic proportions." This is also a good description of how physical disease happens inside your body. If you allow the environment to be created internally for disease, then the mechanisms to create a perfect storm can be assembled. Even in the current cancer research arena, it seems that the answer lies not in winning the war with cancer, but in preventing it. The best answer lies in not creating the environment that would allow cancer to develop in the first place.

If you are having difficulty managing your weight, you are not alone. What is going on with what has become the majority of people in our society? People gain weight, then lose weight, then gain weight back, and then lose it again. First of all, they create a problem situation, because (not being careful) they end up losing weight and then are not gaining back the same type of weight. The scale goes down, and they feel like they did something good. The problem is in most diet situations, people lose muscle, bone, and even internal organ mass. Without intending to, they keep all their fat during the diet. As soon as they stop the diet, they begin to gain back even more weight as fat, but they don't replace the necessary tissues which were lost. Now the situation is even worse in that it becomes harder and harder to lose weight. The composition of the body has been altered and therefore so has its function. Now you can less effectively metabolize fat, experience health, or lose weight.

The truth is that diets just don't work. People don't fail during dieting; the diets fail the people. I will say this again: in my experience, I have found that how much you eat is not nearly as important as what you choose to eat. When people make the right choices by eating proper, real foods, they can easily maintain their health and a proper weight. However, when people eat what most people are eating, they gain excess weight as fat. Real food promotes real results for wellness and weight control. Fake and processed foods promote dysfunction. This leads to people who may even appear skinny yet are actually fat if you consider their body composition and their functional health. Studies done on the most popular diets demonstrate an overall weight loss of only ten pounds. All that money and all that effort, for only ten pounds? That's disappointing, especially if you consider that most end up proportionally fatter than they started.

There are so many different ways to lose weight. The question is, do we want to lose weight in a way that brings us closer to health, or do we simply want the scale to change and indicate a lower number? Many people use fasting or starvation as a way to lose weight. Although an occasional fast might have some health benefits, fasting for weight loss usually is a huge mistake. First of all, when you fast, or even cut back calories too severely, your body will go into that famine response. That means that you will produce ketone bodies but also catabolic products of protein from muscles and organs, you will reset your thyroid and other glands, and good tissue will degrade, accompanied by severe electrolyte imbalances and muscle atrophy. Famine physiology is characterized by a reduced metabolic rate and intense cravings for fatty and carbohydrate-rich foods. In a prolonged famine, you will see increased cortisol, triglycerides, cholesterol, and inflammatory cytokines, and insulin resistance is created. Most damage stems from the loss of active, healthy tissues.

Therefore, as a result of fasting, you will reset your entire physiology in response, and you teach your body to store fat even more efficiently than before. Besides that, you are now less able to maintain your weight or utilize your fat stores for energy. I do not recommend fasting for weight loss unless it is carefully planned, and this is where you may need to consult a practitioner. These controlled fasts are used as a tool for detoxification, seizure control, or creating a very lean body, but we use a carefully planned, protein-sparing modified fast.[1]

---

1 Ketogenic diets can be used to benefit health if the diet is designed correctly. Johns Hopkins and other institutions have used ketogenic fasts for many years, especially to control seizures.
These diets are also used to treat cancer and delay dementia. Many bodybuilders and fitness models can get very lean utilizing this method. If you wish to explore ketogenic strategies, do some research to design the diet to be only beneficial. I will have a future course available on my website at (www.recklesshealth.com).

The famine response is responsible for our survival when food is scarce. It was not intended as a tool for weight loss, and it is not the best way to create health, fitness, or beauty. Your whole body will adapt and reset itself, even creating a different balance of hormones. This is just one example of how you affect an adaptation, which changes how your body works. There are in fact so many ways that you affect the way your body works. In response to any stress, your body adapts and you will be left with the results, whether they are positive or negative. If you pay attention, then you can create adaptations that are beneficial to you. On the other hand, if you're not careful, the change created by adaptation may have consequences that you did not expect or desire.

Instead of fasting, you could try a low-fat diet. Although you might lose weight with this diet, it has been responsible for numerous mental and physical problems. You need the essential fats, and you end up in a very unhealthy state if these are not provided in your diet. When people avoid fats, they tend to eat more sugar in its place. Fats give food their taste, texture, and consistency. Low-fat diets create more inflammation and a poor hormone-balance status, and impact the cardiovascular, reproductive, immune, and nervous systems. Without adequate fats, you cannot manufacture or repair cell plasma membranes, and this is extremely important for proper function. Without a good cell plasma membrane, the cells cannot obtain optimum nutrition, expel harmful waste products, or even maintain fluid balance.

Also, without the *right* fats for your cells, the cells will not function correctly. Hormone receptors, antibodies, and diffusion channels in the cell membrane will be unable to function because you have changed the characteristics of the cell wall. There is even what is termed the "tsunami effect," where improper fats being placed in the cell membrane make it stiff and susceptible to a wave, just like a tsunami. When the wave occurs, the cell wall can be destroyed or least disrupted. A low-fat diet that includes enough essential fats could possibly be a tool to improve your health. Some people are absorbers of fats, while others more efficiently manufacture fats, especially related to cholesterol levels. For people who absorb their fats more readily, a low-fat diet that maintains the intake of good fats can be beneficial. It is all in the details and how the diet is designed.

The production of prostaglandins is also influenced by the type of fats eaten. Prostaglandins regulate body functions such as heart rate, blood pressure, blood clotting, fertility, and conception; play a role in immune function by regulating inflammation; and encourage the body to fight infection. Proper growth in children is dependent on good fat intake, —particularly for neural development and maturation of sensory systems, with male children having even higher need than females—. Many important processes rely on dietary fat intake. There are good functional laboratory tests of biomarkers that can tell us how the systems are working, as well as what can be done to correct any dysfunction. If you have questions about the function of your body, locate a functional medicine practitioner. By learning about function, we avoid many diseases.

You could try a high-protein diet, except that now we need to be concerned about the lack of fiber, a heavier workload for the kidneys, and missing phytonutrients from the lack of plants in our diet. The high-protein diet can be effective for healthy weight loss in the short term—again, if designed properly. I have utilized high-protein diets as treatment, but for the long-term a good ratio and balance of the micronutrients turns out to work the best. There is a great deal of positive research concerning the Mediterranean diet closer to its original form. There is also good research on hunter-gatherer-type diets. It seems that the best and most effective plan is to consume a diet that we have evolved with. What your ancestors ate will probably work out better for you. What we do know is that anyone who consumes primarily processed food products will create a body that cannot work as well.

It is very important to remember that muscle dictates your metabolism. Muscle has the highest density of mitochondria and is a very active tissue of production. Mitochondria are where fat is utilized at the highest rate, and where energy is produced. To be healthy, we need a large amount of active metabolic tissue, good mitochondrial function, and adequate nutrients. Bone cells and fat cells are also very active metabolically. More than targeting loss of weight, we want to target the loss of excess body fat. If not, we end up fatter proportionately, and our fat cells create hormonal and chemical imbalances, as they are proportionately imbalanced in our body composition. If we infiltrate our active tissues (muscle, bone, internal organs) with fat, then they stop working, and this happens as we accumulate more fats. If we have less active tissues and the wrong proportions, then the body cannot function as designed.

There are some crazy, wacky diets that take losing weight to an extreme. Presently the most popular diet of all is the prescription-drug diet. It sounds so simple: just pop a pill and look like a model. The majority of the time this pill will remove our appetite, increase our metabolism, or interfere with body processes that might allow more calories to enter the body. With no appetite, we end up fasting or starving. Why not just lock yourself in a room with no food? You can accomplish the same thing without damaging your body with medication. Drugs may give apparent results because you lose weight, but this is not without the price of side effects and perhaps even permanent damage to your body.

There are diets based entirely on supplements. Okay, instead of taking drugs, you will just take a nutritional or herbal supplement that has the same effect as a medication. Perhaps you purchase pre-prepared meals and take vitamin pills. This will not take the place of good, fresh food, but it will probably lead to weight loss. In some cases, this may help you get started, and with a good plan it might be appropriate. If you're wealthy, and you have someone prepare healthy meals for you, I say go ahead. For most people, there will come a time when we will have to take care of ourselves. There is no better plan than to learn what real food is and to consume just that. Simply taking pills, drinking shakes, applying creams, and all the other shortcuts that people search for will never be as effective in the long term as living and maintaining a better lifestyle.

The low-carbohydrate or no-carbohydrate approach to dieting is used often, and again, it can get people on the right track if it's done correctly. If you consume primarily vegetables, some fruit, and adequate protein, then you have created an effective low-carbohydrate diet. But why work so hard to stay away from carbohydrates if they have benefits for us? I don't want you to minimize carbohydrates to the point that you only eat proteins and fats. This might work for a short time; however, a better strategy is a plan that would ensure that you don't deplete the body of key beneficial nutrients. With low carbohydrate intake, physical and mental performance may suffer, cravings often increase, and mood or emotional disorders ensue. Remember that there are beneficial sources of carbohydrates, like vegetables.

In short, I encourage you to get off the roller coaster of dieting. If you're not careful in your planning, you will lose muscle and then gain fat back in its place. If you continue on, then you will lose more muscle and gain back even more fat. It doesn't take long before you're fatter than you ever were before, even though you weigh the same or less. Is this any way to create a picture of health? Remember, a healthy body, working correctly, will not accumulate any excess fat. A better indicator of health is your body composition. Your weight can be a general guideline; however, measuring the percentage of you that is fat is much more telling and accurate. Currently the BMI (body mass index) is used as a measure of obesity, and this is a relatively simple measurement of body proportion. But a much better measure is the percentage of your body that is composed of fat versus other tissues.

How Our Body Works

To lose weight, we don't need steely determination or military-style discipline. The answer lies in learning how your body works and supporting its systems and mechanisms. The more information you have, the better decisions you can make. If you understand your blood sugar response, you will know how to keep your insulin effective and what affects sugar levels in your blood. You will understand that making better food and physical activity choices are often the entire solution to dangerous conditions like diabetes. We will discuss your body's response to sugar in detail in chapter

4. Carbohydrates can be a tool for physical success, or they can become a weapon of destruction. You may not believe me now; however, as you start to eat more healthy foods and feel better, it becomes very easy to pass up sugary food and drinks.

The human body is really a collection of biological systems. These systems do not work independently of each other and are so integrated that something affecting one system will actually affect them all. Groups of organs, physical structures, organelles, organisms, enzymes, hormones, cytokines, prostaglandins, and other molecules work together, allowing you to be alive. You are a biological-system community, and at the same time, like an orchestra, you do need a conductor to manage the musical score. You are that conductor of the orchestra. The quality of the symphony is directly related to the quality of your lifestyle.

Just so you're aware of what sections you're conducting, the major systems of the body are:

- The circulatory system, delivering blood so that oxygen, nutrients, and messenger molecules arrive at the right place at the right time
- The digestive system, which breaks down, processes, and absorbs nutrients, while at the same time protects the body from foreign substances and parasites through a process of detecting, filtering, and killing
- The endocannabinoid system of neural modulatory lipids and receptors, which regulate appetite, pain, mood, coordination, and memory
- The endocrine system, producing hormones as messengers that trigger specific actions in the body
- The excretory system, removing waste from the body
- The immune system, defending the body against disease-causing agents with immune cells, tonsils, adenoids, thymus, and spleen
- The integumentary system of skin, hair, fat, and nails
- The lymphatic system, involved with the collection and transport of waste products and other molecules

- The muscular system, providing energy, enzymes, and locomotion. This includes smooth muscles that allow arteries in the digestive tract and the respiratory tract to function.
- The nervous system. consisting of the brain, spinal cord, peripheral nervous system, and an ever-changing neural network
- The reproductive system, consisting of the sex organs
- The respiratory system, consisting of the pharynx, larynx, trachea, bronchi, lungs, and diaphragm
- The skeletal system, giving structural support with bones, cartilage, ligaments, and tendons, and producing blood cells and other stem cells
- The urinary system, made up of the kidneys, ureter, bladder, and urethra, which allows fluid balance and electrolyte balance, as well as the excretion of urine

These are the major systems, but there are also minor systems and an infinite number of connections and sharing between the systems. So, all in all, we are a collection of biological systems, and depending on the function being described, we will utilize certain systems of the group. The common thread is that, like an orchestra, we are dependent on every instrument. One instrument "out of tune" or even playing too loud will ruin the entire symphony. Wellness requires a balanced pattern of function. I have listed below some of the tools that you can use as a conductor of your orchestra.

Epigenetics

Let's start with *epigenetics.* Genetics is no longer a science that says genes predetermine everything in your life. Your genetics are now viewed primarily as a source of information, very much like a huge and very comprehensive reference book. How you reference and then use the information contained there is, in so many ways, up to you. As much as 80 percent of the adaptive response that creates phenotypic results is based on your lifestyle. A *phenotype* is the total composite of an organism's observable characteristics or traits. Traits such as morphology, development, biochemical or physiological properties and responses, and behavior and the products of your behavior all become your adaptive response. Your phenotype is the end result of your genetic expression—literally how you look, how you feel, and your experience of disease or wellness. It is, in essence, how your body responds to your lifestyle choices through referencing your book of life (aka your DNA) to produce a result that is based upon the information contained therein. In other words, you direct the eventual outcome, or your genetic expression, in order to fill your lifestyle demands. Your influence is that great in producing your phenotype. You influence your genetic expression through your choices to provide nutrients or not, activity or not, and environmental exposure or not.

It behooves you to become a student of epigenetics. In fact, how your ancestors read their book of life (i.e., their DNA or genomic data) is passed on to you just as much as the genetic information itself: how your ancestors led their lives and adapted to their environment has impacted your genetic expression and that of your progeny. You can choose to repeat their experience (your family history) or you can also choose your own lifestyle and create a different result. Those who came before you survived because they adapted. Some of those adaptations may not be appropriate for today, and others may give you a distinct advantage. How you look, the impact of disease, your behavior, and your experiences are heavily influenced by your own lifestyle, as well as your predecessors. There are more choices and information available to you every day to manage this system as current genomic research moves forward.

Scientists know that they must take into account the effect of lifestyle upon the genetic information. *Epi* means above or around, and *epigenetics* is the study of how different factors change or influence genetic expression. If there is a disease in your family history, that does not mean that you will automatically experience the same disease. If you live your life differently, you are causing a different influence on your genetics, and you will get a different result.

There are recorded cases and studies where even the addition of a single factor can create a different animal. In a study on mice, the single nutrient folate, given to the mother, changed what was expected to be a litter of mice with white fur and with a tendency toward obesity, diabetes and disease, to a litter produced with some babies having dark colored fur, leaner and less susceptible to diseases. In a sense, these were different mice from those that had been bred and what had been expected.

The same concept applies to us. I may have a tendency toward diabetes and obesity, but applying just a few extra elements can make me a completely different person—i.e., healthy and disease resistant.

Allostasis

Allostasis is a science analyzing the effect of stress, based on the understanding that stress is acting upon you all the time. The secret of success is to learn how to use stress for benefit and not to allow it to cause degeneration or maladaptation. Allostasis will cause you to be bigger, faster, stronger, smarter, better functioning, and therefore healthier, if it is applied in the right way. On the other hand, allostasis can be the source for your degenerative demise. The sum total of the stresses you experience is often referred to as the "allostatic load." Stress is both mental and physical, being anything that pushes you off balance. When stress reaches a certain threshold by type or amount, it can cause positive adaptation. Physical therapists study the science of allostasis extensively and can guide a severely injured person back into normal healthy function. When stress is too much, or perhaps when you are not ready for it, there will be a maladaptation, leading to dysfunction and disease.

Triage

In clinical nutrition, scientists are exploring the body's ability to perform *triage*. Because there may be limits to nutrient resources available in your body, priorities must be set. The system of setting priorities was called triage because of the system designed by the French in World War I. *Triage* is a French word meaning "to prioritize." In the stress of the battlefield, when the number of wounded soldiers was overwhelming personnel and local available resources, how do you decide who lives and who dies? Some soldiers with mortal injuries would be euthanized to end their suffering, since there was no way to save their lives. Other soldiers had injuries that required attention, but they could be safely attended to at a later time. Yet others among the wounded, if attended to quickly, could be saved and even perhaps returned to service.

I'm sure you have experienced triage in many situations in your life. When someone else was given priority over you, a critical decision was made about you first. Perhaps you were waiting for a service, and you noticed someone else being attended to before you, even though you had come earlier. Dr. Bruce Ames and other researchers have observed the same mechanism occurring in the human body. The body may often be in a triage situation nutritionally when you do not provide the right balance of nutrients. Your body will try to find within itself the nutrients that it requires, usually by breaking down existing tissues. When physiology cannot find enough nutrients to function, then the body is left with the critical decision of how to keep you alive, but not necessarily how to keep you healthy. Short the supply of important nutrients, and your body will triage, or prioritize a way to sustain your life. The answer may be to shut some biological systems down, or even shunt nutrients from one process to another, destroying optimal function but allowing survival.

Hormones

In our clinic, we work very hard to help people restore hormone balance. This is accomplished through testing current hormone levels in blood, saliva, or urine, and then working to restore ratios and the balance of the different hormones. Next we improve their situation by giving people additional naturally configured hormones, improving their own production of hormones, and correcting the metabolic breakdown of hormones. We also work to improve overall functioning and composition of their bodies.

What you do in life and your state of health directly affects your hormones. You are the key to the proper physiological levels of hormones and how those hormones work together. For example, go on a starvation diet, and you will reset your thyroid gland and the production and conversion of thyroid hormones. Exercise, and you produce additional testosterone and growth hormone to rebuild tissue. Your hormones are messengers trying to keep up with and orchestrate function, according to your demands. You will need hormones for the rest of your life. Hormones like estrogen and progesterone do a lot more than just create the female menstrual cycle. These hormones in particular protect the circulatory system and the nervous system—and, in their normal form and at the correct physiological levels, are actually protective against cancer.

Neurotransmitters

What about your neurotransmitters? Again, these are dependent on the balance of your nutrient intake, food choices, and your overall lifestyle. For example, serotonin, a neurotransmitter often discussed because of its connection to moods and emotions, is actually produced to a great extent in the digestive tract. Because its production is dependent upon the health of your digestive tract, you have the most control over where and when serotonin is produced. Many drugs have been formulated to reduce the uptake and destruction of old serotonin; however, the better choice is to produce fresh serotonin and replenish instead of recycle.

In fact, you have a great deal of control over both the amount of various neurotransmitters produced and how well they will function in the body. You also influence the production of nerves and their myelination. Just like hormones, you will need neurotransmitters for the rest of your life.

Xenohormesis

Xenohormesis is a process of communication between the body and things outside it in its environment. Xenohormesis is demonstrated when a very small amount of something produces a much larger than expected effect (i.e., a hormetic effect). The process of xenohormesis is described in several studies where plants have been found to communicate important information to the human body. The severity of the weather and other stresses in the environment of the plant are actually communicated to the human body when the plant is eaten. Substances produced by the plant even in very small amounts stimulate the body to respond in anticipation of events the plant adapted to. It is an early warning system as well as an inducing force for the body to prepare for current environmental conditions. This is one of the reasons why we talk about eating local, seasonal foods. This xenohormetic effect can be positive, in the case of small molecules in broccoli such as DIM, which can positively influence how estrogen is metabolized and prevent cancer, or sulforaphane, which has anticancer, antidiabetic, and antimicrobial properties. This effect can also be negative, when a small amount of something toxic causes a negative disease response, even death.

Being overweight is a sign of dysfunction, and the problem is much larger internally than what appears outwardly. In my experience, people who consume whole, real foods do not have a weight problem, and they experience a healthier life. The food you choose is communication to your body. Proper communication creates proper function, and this in turn creates wellness.

It is after all, you, who chooses whatever you put into your mouth. If you eat real food, then you automatically end up practicing caloric restriction. The calories will take care of themselves, since the proportion of nutrients is much higher. Generally caloric restriction exists when calories are reduced 10-30 percent.

Society, and even doctors, have gotten into the habit of practicing medicine like the armchair quarterback on the day after the game. Medicine has become "after the fact" diagnosis and treatment. It is dealing with the animals who ran away again by examining the open barn door after the fact but never closing the door in the first place. If you learn about prevention and you enhance physiological function, you can prevent the occurrence of the disease. In conventional medicine, prevention in most cases is simply discovering a fulminant disease early. Then treatment protocols are applied to symptoms and you remain under disease management of some kind. In functional medicine, we focus on the triggers and causes of dysfunction so that we can minimize symptoms and avoid the outcome of the disease itself. If you restore function and understand mechanisms, the body can operate very well without the interference.

Disease is not all up to chance and fate; it is primarily developed through lifestyle choices. There is a mechanism to every disease that you ever experience. Everything has to be in place for the disease to start and for it to progress. Living a congruent lifestyle means eating the food and using the body in a way and in an environment that it has adapted to. The body is always doing what it is supposed to do. It is up to us to place it in situations that it can handle. If it cannot, we will have to adapt it ourselves so that it can.

Your Plan to Create Health and Prevent Disease

Let's create a new plan together. I am going to give you a plan for absolute, vibrant health. There are four major areas that you have control of in our lifestyle plan. This book is laid out in four parts that discuss each area of the plan in detail.

Part One: Eat Real Food is about food and nutrients, our first tool. In order to create health, eat real food. The food-like substances that most of us consume hardly bear any resemblance to the actual food that they came from. In modern society, we don't consume whole grains; we tend to consume grain products like flour. We don't consume healthy animals; we consume feedlot, fenced, and caged animals who did not consume the foods that they were designed for. We don't consume vegetables, unless you count lettuce, pickles, and ketchup. Our food is canned, packaged, genetically modified, and laced with chemical pesticides and preservatives. We voluntarily eat them and expect to be well.

Part Two: Get Physically Active concerns physical activity. The body is designed to move. When we are sedentary, biological systems begin to shut down and tissues atrophy and are lost. Energy production is impaired and lessened. Circulation is impaired. The nerves shrink and become dysfunctional. Without adequate exercise, the process of aging and degeneration is accelerated. The upside is that the body can regenerate as well. This is driven by physical activity. Your body adapts by responding to imposed demands, like activity.

Part Three: Detoxify is a discussion of detoxification. When you allow an accumulation, or "body burden," of substances in the body, this interferes with the function of the body. Many symptoms can be attributed to this "burden," since symptoms occur only when the body is in dysfunction. Cleanse the body to remove some of the burden, and things just work better.

Part Four: Stress and the Healthy Mind deals with our response to stress. When we understand stress, we can use it for our advantage and even create adaptations. If we just allow stress to have its effect, we often suffer maladaptation and sustain injury.

With a lifestyle plan in place, you will have little or no need for a health plan. Insurance and the whole medical complex are well equipped in the emergency setting. They do an excellent job of dealing with trauma and treating acute disease. However, there is a real lack of effective management for chronic mental and physical disorders. I suggest that you don't get sick, and I am not kidding.

Part One

Eat Real Food

It Comes Naturally

Chapter 2

The Case for Real Food

Quality Is More Important than Quantity

What is "real food?" What are we talking about here? Over thousands of years, your body has evolved along with and become accustomed to using certain substances as a source of energy, nutrients, and hormetic molecules. Identifiable foods tend to come from our environment and are usually most beneficial for us with a minimum of preparation or tampering. For the sake of convenience in our society, we have adopted the use of processed food substances. As a general rule, the more that you process, alter, and package a food, the less value it has for you as a human being. In fact, many things intentionally added to the food to change its normal characteristics are harmful by themselves. Recently it has also been discovered that things in the packaging of food also taint our food.

If you enter many modern supermarkets, it may even be hard to find anything identifiable as the original food. I have visited supermarkets where the produce section was smaller than an average bedroom, though the building contained several thousand square feet of packaged "convenience" foods. Dr. Barry Sears in his book *The Zone* talks about shopping the perimeter of the supermarket, where the produce, fresh proteins, and relatively unaltered foods are displayed. It is interesting that if you venture into the center of most supermarkets, you will find packages that have to be labeled as food, otherwise you would not know if they were edible or not.

Now before I tread any further, let's get one thing straight. I understand fully that we live in a modern age, with foods redesigned for convenience, shelf life, taste, and availability. I am not writing this intending that you will never eat a slice of bread or enjoy cake, candy, cookies, or your favorite treats. What I am proposing is that the majority of the time you consume actual, identifiable, health-promoting foods. Please consider the degree to which each food is healthy for you and will enhance function, most of the time. If a piece of bread looks white, quite uniform, and just melts in your mouth, it is primarily starch. Don't consider this good nutrition, but if as one your favorite foods bread is enjoyed occasionally, that is quite acceptable. I am proposing that if you consume bread, it should at least have some fiber content (somewhere around 8 grams per slice) and that you can identify whole or pieces of grains, nuts, or seeds.

Just because the label says "whole wheat" does not mean that it is any more than a dark-colored starch. Compare what the food was originally to what it looks like now. Have chemicals been added, like pesticides to deter insects or preservatives to ensure packaged food has a better shelf life? How altered is the food from its original state? Whole-wheat bread tends to be nothing more than brown flour, and it is not a whole-grain product. Grains are intact grains and usually need to be slightly cooked to be more edible. Most people consume grains as a flour product with food coloring, added sugar, and in different shapes, making them more about marketing than proper nutrition. This includes most breakfast cereals.

"Real food" is just what it says: foods that come direct from the farmer or rancher who raised them as much as possible. You have to ask some critical questions and understand what happened before it is in your hands. Was the food raised naturally, or was it protected with pesticides and modified for yield but not for nutritional value? You may be eating a genetically modified food, which has altered proteins and can do harm to humans and other animals fed with it. These animals may then even harm the humans that consume them. Many plants produce more beneficial nutrients if the plants themselves grow in an environment that is natural. When the plants are stressed by wind, rain, sun, and other aspects of the environment, they actually become more nutritious for us, as they produce their own stress chemicals. When your only objective is high yield or pest resistance, the actual plants hold much less nutritional value. When organically grown foods are tested, they actually do have a higher nutrient content because they were allowed to grow normally.

If you consume animals and animal products, do you know if the animal was fed the food that it has evolved to eat and was therefore a healthy animal? Many animals that we consume are fed things that shorten that animal's lifespan. There are animal feeds that the animal was not designed to eat, like grains, silage, and animal byproducts. Some cows bred for consumption actually feed on dead animals and waste products, when cows are designed to eat grass. An herbivore needs to stick with its natural food. Cows that are fed unnatural diets, supplemented with antibiotics and hormone growth factors, are different animals altogether. The structure of the protein of their meat is altered, and the type and content of fat is much different. Grass-fed beef—animals that were raised naturally—actually have a protein structure and fat content that are healthy for human consumption. The studies showing health consequences from consumption of red meat really demonstrate the fact that we need to become more aware of whether we are consuming healthy animals or not.

The studies do not show that the consumption of naturally raised animals or especially wild-game red meat is harmful. In fact, studies done on healthier animals, such as grass-fed beef, show that it is healthy to consume and actually contains the unsaturated fats that we try to get people to take supplements for. In fact, there was a study in Australia comparing wild kangaroo meat consumption with the consumption of grain-fattened cattle. Markers of inflammation and other poor health indicators were completely different, being higher in the human subjects who consumed the unnatural fattened cattle. People were healthier, depending on the type of meat consumed. Other studies have also demonstrated that we can benefit from even red meat if the animal itself was healthy. There has never been a healthy cow or other animal that was raised on silage and grain.

Vegetables themselves offer a great deal more value when consumed as real food. The best way to consume vegetables is with minimum preparation, ideally raw or steamed. I come in contact with so many clients who don't like the taste of vegetables or find them inconvenient to prepare. Then there's the person who believes their vegetable intake will be adequate if they just eat some lettuce and tomato once in a while. I consider tomatoes to be a fruit anyway, and lettuce, at least the iceberg form, does not hold a great deal of value. Studies indicate that people who consume as many as ten servings of vegetables or more per day tend to be much healthier. I hope this is a joke: please don't count the ketchup as a serving of vegetables. Bear in mind that a vegetable serving is about a cupful raw.

Currently most nutritionists are recommending at least five servings and as many as thirteen servings of vegetables per day. If you currently get none, I suggest that you start with one serving per day. Then you can slowly work up cup by cup. Be aware that there are different colors of vegetables (green, red, purple, orange, blue, and white), and ideally they would be consumed practically every day. If a serving is about a cup of raw vegetables, we are literally talking about as many as thirteen cups of vegetables consumed every day. A variety of color on your plate is just as important since different colors provide different nutrients giving you the variety that you will benefit from.

I am not a strong proponent of juicing, green drinks, vegetable chips, or several of the other ways people have found to "increase vegetable

Green	Red	Purple/Blue	Orange/Yellow	White
Vegetables	*Vegetables*	*Vegetables*	*Vegetables*	*Vegetables*
Artichokes	Beet	Black salsify	Butternut	Cauliflower
Arugula	Radicchio	Eggplant	squash	Garlic
Asparagus	Radishes	Purple Belgian	Carrots	Ginger
Broccoflower	Red bell pepper	endive	Rutabagas	Jerusalem
Broccoli	Red chili	Purple potatoes	Sweet corn	artickoke
Broccoli rabe	peppers	Purple asparagus	Sweet potatoes	Jicama
Brussel sprouts	Red onions	Purple cabbage	Yellow beets	Kohlrabi
Celery	Red peppers	Purple carrots	Yellow peppers	Mushrooms
Chayote squash	Red potatoes	Purple peppers	Yellow potatoes	Parsnips
Chinese cabbage	Rhubarb		Yellow summer	Potatoes
Cucumber		*Fruits*	squash	Shallots
Endive	*Fruits*	Purple figs	Yellow winter	Turnips
Green beans	Tomatoes	Purple grapes	squash	White corn
Green cabbage	Watermelon	Raisins		Onions
Green onion	Strawberries	Black currants	*Fruits*	
Green pepper	Red pear	Blackberries	Cape	*Fruits*
Leafy greens	Blood orange	Blueberries	Gooseberries	Bananas
Leeks	Raspberries	Dried plums	Golden kiwifruit	Brown pears
Lettuce	Grapefruit	Elderberries	Grapefruit	Dates
Okra		Grapes	Lemon	White
Peas		Plums	Mangoes	Nectarines
Snow peas		Pomegranates	Nectarines	White peaches
Spinach		Prunes	Oranges	
Sugar snap peas			Papayas	
Watercress			Peaches	
Zucchini			Persimmons	
Fruits			Pineapples	
Avocados			Pumpkin	
Green apples			Tangerines	
Green grapes			Yellow apples	
Green pears			Yellow figs	
Kiwifruit			Yellow pears	
			Yellow tomatoes	
			Yellow	
			watermelon	
			Apricots	
			Cantaloupe	

intake," although this is better than nothing at all. Although I often recommend using vegetable juice for cancer support, this is an entirely different situation. If I am working with somebody and their oncologist to help them survive cancer and its treatment, then I need to use nutrients, and even vegetables, just like I would use medication or drugs. If we juice vegetables, we get a very high concentration of the phytonutrients. I want this high concentration to stimulate, induce, and protect the person who is dealing with cancer. We will also use higher doses of nutrients like vitamins, minerals, and other compounds.

In a normal, healthy person, the concentration of these chemical phytonutrients, and especially sugars, can actually become too high of a dose. Some very helpful nutrients in plants when taken in a small dosage are very health promoting. A number of things in plants have a hormetic effect, where a small amount of the chemical can produce a large response. So for the average person, it is best to consume a reasonable amount of vegetables in their whole form. If I'm trying to treat a disease, then I may use a higher concentration in the same way that I might use a pharmaceutically developed chemical; otherwise, the body is designed to digest real food and intact fiber, and extract and absorb the nutrients that it needs.

Fruits also contain valuable nutrients; however, they also tend to contain a fair amount of sugar, especially tropical fruits. If we look at the total amount of valuable nutrients, fruits come in second to vegetables. That is why the current recommendation for fruit intake is only two to four servings a day, while the recommended vegetable intake is up to thirteen servings. I don't mean to say that we should not consume fruit; however, it is better to have a higher ratio of vegetables, perhaps three times the intake of fruit.

Legumes, beans, nuts, and seeds are valuable as well. Even though vegetables contain fats, many of the nuts and seeds are an even better source for the essential fats that we require. Many legumes also contain a fair amount of protein, although many of the beans are also carbohydrates, which should be kept in mind. We also have to consider some of the natural chemicals in beans, which may be hard on the body.

The processing and preparation of food is best if it is minimized. The primary reason for cooking food is perhaps to aid digestion, but more importantly to sterilize a food that might be unsafe. We cook food to minimize exposure to bacteria, virus, and parasites. But the cooking of food also changes its characteristics and its nutritional value. The more that you cook a protein, the more you alter its form and the less valuable it is for you. Proteins become denatured and altered in their structure. When you overcook animal proteins and fats, they can become altered to a point where they are carcinogenic. Overcooked or well-done meat contains advanced glycation end products, which will be discussed later in the book, as well as chemicals formed by the heating process.

Even though soup stocks, especially those containing bone, can have health benefits, when you cook especially vegetables too much, you also alter and lose some of the beneficial nutrients. Enzymes and other nutrients are destroyed, and some nutrients are even thrown out when the liquid is not consumed. Fresh-frozen vegetables still retain most of the benefits. However, the canning process starts with overcooking, and even in modern-day canning, the plastics that line the can and the lead or other substances that seal it can leach into the food and destroy health benefits.

The ideal situation would be one where we all had the time and the space to produce our own food. We'd know exactly how it was raised, what chemicals it was exposed to, and what was done to it before we consumed it. In our modern world, this is just not practical anymore. Most of us are dependent on specialization and industrialization. The only source we have for the food that we consume is outside of our control. However, you still have the power to choose healthy food. You also can refuse to buy and consume the food-like substances that are processed beyond recognition. Whether you frequently purchase your food from the supermarket or consume most of your meals at a restaurant, there will always be good choices and poor choices.

I encourage you to make the more beneficial choice most of the time. Real food can be convenient, especially with a little forethought. Every one of your meals does not have to be prepackaged; it is well worth preparing a few of your own. If you eat frequently at another place of business, then choose an eating establishment that also values your health. Most eating establishments are more than happy to serve you healthier choices. It should not be a problem to exchange an item from your plate for something healthier in its place. Perhaps instead of the fries, you get another serving of vegetables.

It is well worth investigating, if you can, a little about the diet that your ancestors consumed. You have also evolved to consume a similar diet to theirs. Dr. Weston Price spent a great deal of time studying indigenous peoples and paid close attention to the foods that they consumed. He had expected to find that without the conveniences of modern civilization, these people would be in a poor state of health. After all, they did not have modern doctors and dentists or the benefit of modern science. They were continuing to eat what they had always eaten, and to live the way they had for generations.

In his book *Nutrition and Physical Degeneration,* he describes what he found. It was the opposite of his original conclusions. He found that people who consumed the natural diets of their societies tended to be very healthy and did not suffer the major diseases of Western civilization. They contended with cuts and bruises and broken bones. They did not have to deal with cancer, heart disease, diabetes, depression, and the whole list of chronic diseases Western civilization contends with. As a dentist, he observed perfect teeth and gums in these people.

Dr. Price demonstrated how these peoples were healthy in their native habitat. He also observed that when they started to consume a more modern, Western-civilization-type diet and adopt that lifestyle, they would contract our modern diseases. In societies with literally no reported Western diseases, these problems would begin to appear. He even tried to explain depression to the Eskimos, and they could not conceive of a situation where a person could become dysfunctional in their life from a mental problem. In their society, inactivity meant certain death. The only thing that they could relate to that was even close to depression was grieving when someone was lost. I encourage you to explore his book. There are other authors who confirm his observations.

Your body was adapted to an ancestral diet, and the closer you stay to this original eating plan, likely the better you will feel and the better your body will function. The original Mediterranean diet has been well studied scientifically. In recent studies, it has been considered to be one of the healthiest diets in modern times. Consider that these studies were also performed on people who share that ancestry. The Asian diet is also looked at as one of the healthier diets. The consistent theme shared by most of these diets is the consumption of fresher, unprocessed foods and the minimization of high calorie intake.

Our modern American diet has been proven to be associated with, and even has become a causative factor in, many current chronic diseases and conditions. There is likely no one who is suited to eat what many in this country eat today. For a number of people, it has become a diet consisting entirely of flour: Cold cereal in the morning (which is essentially sugar, flour, and food coloring) macaroni and cheese for lunch, and noodles or spaghetti for dinner. (We'll talk more about the effects of this kind of diet in later chapters.) The consumption of vegetables, good quality protein, and unsaturated fats are almost forgotten components. How can you expect to build and maintain a healthy body and mind with this type of diet?

Remember, obesity and weight management is not a simple "calories in, calories out" equation. As a person begins to accumulate fat, the fat itself actually reinforces the dysfunctional situation. Fat cells produce hormones, cytokines, and other substances that reinforce the accumulation of more fat. It's almost as if the fat cells are perpetuating themselves. Many people believe that overweight people experience joint pain and feeling physically and emotionally drained because of the physics of weight and gravity. It is actually the dysfunction created from these chemicals that the fat cells overproduce.

Food is communication, and it always has an effect in the body. What messages are you providing to your body? What you eat sends a message, and there will be a response. That response may not be a positive experience for the body, especially if the immune response is triggered too strongly. When we consume natural and known foods, the immune response is small, even negligible, but usually positive in the scheme of body function. When we consume new-to-nature molecules (drugs and manufactured chemicals), altered proteins and fats, concentrated starches and sugars, and other unnatural items, there is a hyper-immune response from the body, and we feel sick.

Some foods include chemicals that induce our body to function properly for the current environmental conditions through a positive and appropriate hormetic effect, in that it doesn't take a large amount of these chemicals to produce the response. Many plants, when stressed, will produce chemicals that notify our body to be ready for stress and get ready for action when we consume those plants. Some chemicals produced by plants influence how we metabolize certain molecules, like hormones. It is up to you to learn what real food is. Don't be taken in by marketing pictures or descriptions or buzzwords. It is probably better to ignore much of how the product is presented and to pay more attention to what is actually in the package. Just because the package says "whole-grain," "natural," or "organic," or claims some health benefit, it is important that you determine the actual ingredients or contents, and know for yourself that this product will help you maintain your health. Most products probably started out as a nutritious food, but after processing and packaging, they hold much less value for you. With that in mind, here's a list of real foods that should be basic to your diet.

Real Foods List

Vegetables

Probably your best source for carbohydrates is vegetables. They are your best choice to lower calories and to maximize nutrient intake. Plants can be a source for protein and also for good fats (five to thirteen servings recommended each day):

Asparagus, beets, bell peppers, broccoli, brussel sprouts, cabbage, carrots, cauliflower, celery, collard greens, cucumbers, eggplant, fennel, garlic, green beans, green peas, kale, leeks, mushrooms, mustard greens, olives, onions, potatoes, romaine lettuce, sea vegetables, spinach, squash, sweet potato, Swiss chard, turnip greens, yams.

Fruits

Fruits are also primarily carbohydrate but often are not as nutrient dense as vegetables. They are still acceptable (two to four servings recommended each day):

Apples, apricots, bananas, blueberries, blackberries, cantaloupe, cranberries, figs, grapefruit, grapes, kiwi, lemon, lime, orange, papaya, pears, pineapple, plums, prunes, raisins, raspberries, strawberries, tomatoes, watermelon.

Eggs and Dairy

Eggs and dairy contain primarily protein and fats. Their value depends on how the animal was raised. Try to buy "free-range" or grass-fed animal products:

Cheese, eggs, milk, yogurt.

Beans and Legumes

Beans and legumes can be a good source of protein; however, they tend to contain a higher amount of carbohydrates as well:

Black beans, dried peas, garbanzo beans, kidney beans, lentils, lima beans, miso, navy beans, pinto beans, soybeans.

Animal Meats

Animal meats are primarily protein and, depending on how the animals were raised, can contain good fats. The benefit to consuming animals is the ability to consume complete protein along with other nutrients.

Beef (ideally grass fed and organic), chicken, lamb, turkey, venison, bison, other wild game meats.

Seafood

Seafood tends to be the most easily digested and is regarded as a good source of unsaturated fats.

Cod, halibut, salmon, sardines, scallops, shrimp, tuna, herring.

Nuts and Seeds

Nuts and seeds are sources of good fats as well as protein.

Almonds, cashews, flaxseed,[2] extra-virgin cold-processed olive oil, peanut, pumpkin seeds, sesame seeds, sunflower seeds, walnuts.

Whole Grains

Whole grains are best in their unprocessed form, often consumed as a hot cereal. It is also important to know if you are sensitive to gluten or allergic to certain grasses.

Barley, brown rice, buckwheat, corn, millet, oats, quinoa, rye, spelt, wheat.

Herbs and Spices

Herbs and spices are often used to flavor foods and make them more palatable. Studies have shown that many of these also contain powerful chemicals that are beneficial. For example, curcumin is under study because

2 A short note: some studies have indicated that high intake of flax may not be good for males because it may promote prostate disease. Females, though, do very well with flax, and males can benefit from a small amount.

of its major benefit in controlling immune response and even perhaps the treatment of cancer. Cinnamon is very effective to help control blood sugar levels.

Basil, black pepper, cayenne pepper, chili pepper, cilantro, coriander, cinnamon, cloves, curcumin, dill, ginger, mustard seeds, oregano, parsley, peppermint, rosemary, sage, thyme.

Safer Natural Sweeteners

Molasses, honey, maple syrup, agave, stevia.

Just Do It

This list is by no means every food that I would recommend. It is a listing of example foods that should be basic to your diet. Consume them as much as possible so that your body can function and stay healthy. Again, there are occasions where the consumption of nonfood is appropriate. There is absolutely no reason why we can't enjoy occasional baked goods and other treats, especially in the way of celebration. There also might be benefits for a professional bodybuilder or athlete who intends to stimulate an insulin response in order to build muscle faster or become leaner. When the intake is only occasional and you are primarily consuming real food, you will reap the benefits.

If you're still struggling with the concept of real food, please visit my website at www.reckless health.com for more information and print, audio, and video. If you already have a grasp on the information presented here, then I wish you well; go for it. And to borrow a concept from Nike, "JUST DO IT."

Chapter 3

Grains and Dairy

Blessing or Curse?

There is no doubt that you can keep people alive utilizing grains, grain products, and dairy products. In fact, you can feed a lot of people with processed grains and starch, and we do so around the world all the time. It is fairly easy to grow large amounts of grains and process them into several different food-like substances. These "foods" will sustain life and can keep people alive in drought or famine. In fact, many researchers worry that we might not be able to produce enough food for the people of the world without grain products. The question is, do these grain-product foods create a healthy person, or is there something missing? In what form can grains be eaten and still hold value? Can we thrive on these food-like substances, or is it merely survival?

For many people, avoiding grains and/or dairy becomes a much healthier way to live. In fact, the majority of people experience an immune response and other reactions to both grain and dairy products. Some people react so strongly that it is life threatening. For example, people who have celiac disease cannot eat grains because of the damage that gluten does to their intestinal wall. A large number of people cannot tolerate dairy, especially once it is pasteurized and or homogenized. At the same time, there are people who do not produce the enzyme to break down lactose, or the sugar contained in milk.

We know that vegetables carry many nutrients and produce health benefits for us as humans when they are consumed. We know that whole fruits, nuts, and seeds carry in them fiber, oils, and other beneficial nutrients. We can get protein from animals, legumes, and even plants. So the question is, do we really need grain and dairy products? They are prevalent in our culture and some people do fine with them; however, especially once they are processed, they can become a hazard to consume for almost everyone. Gluten can carry inflammation throughout the body, starting in the digestive tract. When processed, dairy products become of much less value to us, as proteins and fats are altered. On the other hand, in some studies, certain components of dairy can be beneficial if correctly processed. For example, whey protein from the liquid portion of milk, if processed cold and then carefully isolated, can be a very beneficial protein source. However, some whey protein is simply dried milk, still containing contaminants and also altered by the processing.

But even the proteins in grains and milk themselves, gluten and casein, can affect you adversely in a number of ways. Many will suffer an allergic response or localized inflammation and then have symptoms as a result. The symptoms are often mild and not given much attention, but they have an additive effect. Many dairy and all gluten products tend to have a higher sugar content, grain products being primarily starch. Starch is sugar, and if you increase your intake of sugar you tend to increase the amount of glycation, abnormal receptors, free radicals, and actual foreign bodies in your blood. Body tissues are damaged and even cholesterol is changed into something that poses danger.

Note: cholesterol normally produced is never dangerous to anyone. However when the cholesterol is glycated, oxidized, and damaged in other ways, cholesterol particle number and size is altered, and at that point the cholesterol produces damage and cardiovascular disease. Also, there is risk when people produce different lipoproteins in the cholesterol. This can all be improved upon with diet and nutrients.

Gluten and casein also cause a drug-like response, as the molecules caseomorphine and gliadomorphine are very similar to opiates and have the same effect on people. The opiates, such as morphine and codeine and several other alkaloids, have side effects such as pulmonary edema, respiratory depression, coma, cardiac, and/or respiratory failure. Some opiates are produced by the body itself, like enkephalins and endorphins. Similar molecules are absorbed in the digestive tract either as medication or components of food, such as casemorphins (from milk), gliadomorphins (from gluten), exorphins, and rubiscolins. Sensitivity to these peptides vary, but they all resemble opiates and act as opiates. The opioid food peptides have links of typically four to eight amino acids. The body's own opioids are generally much longer. Brain opioid peptide systems are known to play an important role in motivation, emotion, attachment behavior, the response to stress and pain, and the control of food intake.

Similar to brain neurotransmitters, gluten and casein's protein structure can interfere with normal neural network function. They may affect weight loss, moods, self-control, depression, focus, and concentration, and they can influence endorphin receptors in the brain, actually becoming addictive.

Grains, Gluten Sensitivity, and Celiac Disease

Unfortunately, in the drive to produce higher yields, pest resistance, higher gluten content, and higher selling value, the food industry has altered grains from their original and natural state. We had actually evolved with wild, harvested grains, and some humans could do very well by consuming the whole grain. But these whole, original, and natural grains are really not available today, and there is good evidence that these new, genetically modified grains can be harmful to us. Genetic modification may allow us to have a grain with higher yield, higher gluten content, and pest resistance; however, the protein and other components have now been altered to something different that our bodies may not accept. Also, the gluten content, being now much higher, has also evidenced itself in more gluten-connected diseases.

On top of that, the form of these grains that most people consume is really highly processed flour, which is no longer a whole grain. You could track the average American's entire diet and see that it is based on flour products. Commonly, we consume a cold cereal in the morning, which is primarily flour, colored and shaped appropriate to the marketing. The cold cereal most people eat in the morning contains virtually no nutritional value except what has been "enriched" or put back in. Much of the nutritional value in the grain is contained in its oil and germ. By the time a grain is ground into flour, most of the nutritional value has been disposed of. We tend to use just the flour. For lunch, we eat macaroni and cheese, or some other flour product like bread or tortillas. At dinner time, perhaps we'll have a big bowl of spaghetti, and then some chips and fake cheese while we watch TV.

Gluten content is also much higher these days, and we know that many people are sensitive to it, suffering an immune response to several glutens, especially those in the Poaceae family (grasses, or monocot flowering plants). The primary grains in this family are wheat, rye, and barley, to name a few. It was thought in the past that very few people were gluten sensitive. However, at that time, the gluten content in our foods was relatively low, so that people were not exposed to as high of a dose. Now with higher gluten content in the grains, more people are reacting simply because of this higher dose.

The bottom line is that grains and grain products are not necessary for health. Our ancestors did not consume many cultivated grains until between 5,000 to 10,000 years ago, and only in some selected societies (China and Egypt). We also have descriptions of some wild harvesting of grains as well. Rice, as a grain, seemed to be the safer alternative over wheat, rye, and barley grasses. Interestingly, there is no strong evidence of cardiovascular disease until Egypt, which was the first society to cultivate wheat. There is a lot more evidence today implicating these cultivated and processed grains as the cause of disease.

For some people, they can be a component of the diet if they are tolerated. Remember that "whole grain" refers to the intact grain eaten, perhaps as a hot cereal. Consider how much the grain product you consume differs from the original whole grain. Are you really getting a good fiber source—for example, looking for 4 to 8 grams or more per slice of bread? Can you see existing grains in whole or in part in the food? If the package says "whole grain," "whole wheat," "natural," or "health," that does not necessarily mean that the bread or the product contains anything more than flour. If you consume grain and grain products, try to apply the whole food concept and steer clear of extensive processing.

A very important measurement to watch is the glycemic index (see the next chapter for more about carbohydrates and the glycemic index). I suggest your major source of carbohydrates should actually come from vegetables and some from fruits. I especially encourage you to not spend your day consuming flour, starch, and sugar.

Gluten Sensitivity and Celiac Sprue

More people than ever before have been identified to have *gluten sensitivity*. Gluten, gliadin, and glutenin are proteins in the grain, which form the protein source destined to feed the sprouting seed. Some people can consume this protein without any reaction or concern. However, with more sensitive testing, the percentage of people who react adversely to this protein is much higher than previously thought. Specifically, the majority of people are found to react to the gluten in the group of plants called monocots. The triticum family in this group contains the most commonly reactive glutens encountered—in wheat, rye, and barley. There are other grains in this family as well, including einkorn, emmer, and variations of wheat, such as durum, semolina, couscous, spelt, and kamut.

Gluten sensitivity can produce a few annoying symptoms, or the reaction can be so extreme that there is permanent damage to the digestive tract (as in celiac sprue, or celiac disease).

When people with gluten sensitivity eat gluten, it causes an inflammatory response. Many patients harbor a gene that increases such an interaction with gluten. The HLA–DQ 2 protein or the HLA–DQ 8 protein are often tested for. These HLA molecules identify gluten fragments that promote the direct attack on the intestinal lining itself. Other genes are likely to be involved as well. In most people, protein links control what are termed "tight junctions" and hold the intestinal cells together. These epithelial (intestinal) cells stand shoulder to shoulder like sentries, acting to filter what is allowed into the bloodstream. In those with celiac disease or more extensive gluten sensitivity, the junctions come apart, allowing a large amount of indigestible gluten fragments and other undigested foods to seep in the underlying tissue and trigger immune system cells.

This leads to a situation of increased permeability in the gut, allowing larger particles to pass through the bloodstream. When any protein sets off an immune response, tissues in the proximity of that protein are also affected. So when gluten gets into the bloodstream, it travels to other regions and creates inflammation there. If this happens in the brain, this can cause Alzheimer's disease and dementia. If the gluten cells end up elsewhere, the localized inflammation can cause damage in that place. Eventually we are seeing higher incidences of autoimmune disease where the inflammatory response is aimed at the host tissue. Literally, your immune system starts to react to you.

With gluten sensitivity, there is good evidence of a direct relationship to cancer, autoimmune disease, osteoporosis, brain disorders, intestinal diseases, chronic pain, digestive disorders, infertility, and problematic pregnancies. The intestinal lining is a significant part of your immune system, and it prevents pathogens, antigens, toxins, and undigested food from entering the bloodstream. If the intestinal lining is damaged, these undesirable substances and organisms will enter the blood much more easily—in addition to the undigested gluten proteins freely circulating in the bloodstream and damaging the remote tissue wherever they end up. If either of these scenarios occur on a regular basis, the chances of developing a serious disease are significantly higher.

For example, it has been our experience in the clinic (and this has now been written up in certain case studies) that there is a strong connection between gluten sensitivity and Hashimoto's thyroiditis. The consumption of gluten seems to mimic thyroid tissue. In many cases, this connection has been so strong that people have developed hypothyroidism. The good news is that we do see thyroid function improve for these people if they avoid gluten and do things to support the thyroid. These people may need thyroid hormone, but the improvement is measurable. There are two types of thyroid antibodies commonly measured, and the avoidance of gluten has a direct effect on reducing those antibodies and improving thyroiditis.

But if left unaddressed, under all this stress, the adrenal glands produce more cortisol in order to reduce the inflammation and ready the body to respond to the situation. When this happens frequently, it will likely lead to adrenal fatigue and in turn cause further problems. Adrenal exhaustion leads to poor sleep, little or no energy, and a body that cannot respond in a way that is supposed to.

In celiac disease, nutritional absorption is also affected. In a normal digestive tract, food is sterilized and digested in the stomach. Then the food enters the intestine lined with fingerlike projections called villi, which, among other things, provides increased surface area for the absorption of nutrients. Enzymes produced by the pancreas and from the epithelial cells continue the breakdown of most of the food into even smaller components such as glucose, amino acids, and other nutrients. Once broken down to small units, these nutrients are allowed to pass into the bloodstream, providing nutrition to the body. In celiac disease, intestinal sites become damaged from the immune response to gluten. When enough damage occurs, this flattens the villi, reducing surface area in the intestine and impairing or even stopping absorption.

What this means is that as a person's intestinal lining sustains damage, they can literally die from malnutrition even when consuming enough food. First they lose the ability to filter nutrients properly and protect the bloodstream from the unwanted things in the digestive tract. This is called a "leaky gut," where there is more permeability. Then when damage has reached a point where there is no path to the blood, absorption is impaired or stops altogether. They cannot absorb nutrients from their food, so they must find other ways to nourish their bodies. At times the situation is so severe we have to give them nutrients in a concentrated liquid form or even through an IV.

If someone has celiac disease, it is imperative that they avoid grains completely, so that this damage does not occur. Even someone who is gluten sensitive is better off if they avoid gluten, since they are producing higher levels of inflammation. As we stated, the situation is further complicated when gluten is able to gain access to the bloodstream because of damage in the intestines and this increased permeability. Now the gluten can travel anywhere in the body carried by the circulation. Wherever the gluten ends up, even in the brain, inflammation will occur as a person reacts to the gluten, and this can become very serious.

Are You Gluten Sensitive?

Are you sensitive to wheat, rye, barley, or any other gluten-containing food? Do you have a weight problem, finding it difficult to lose weight and that you are gaining more weight? Do you often feel bloated? Do you notice swelling in your fingers, ankles, and other joints? Do you find that your mood and behavior are out of your control? These and other signs of an immune-system response very likely are the result of a sensitivity to food. If you're trying to control your weight, eating gluten and processed foods can trigger an immune response, and this will create a weight gain of water simply from the inflammatory response. Headaches, itchy eyes, and many other allergy symptoms are also often exhibited in response to consuming gluten.

In fact, one of the most common reactions to gluten, especially in people with celiac sprue, is a skin condition called dermatitis herpetiformis. I remember a patient who had not been able to feel the bones in her fingers, and she thought her fingers were reacting abnormally to her new diet after we took her off gluten. She had spent her entire life with so much swelling from gluten foods that it alarmed her when her hands were normal and no longer swollen.

It is difficult sometimes to determine food sensitivities because the symptoms are often delayed for hours or days after you consume the food. Commonly, the symptoms appear seventy-two hours later, and symptoms have even been tracked up to two weeks later. An effective and accurate way to determine food sensitivity is to design an elimination diet. For a period of two weeks up to three months, you consume a diet that does not include any of the food suspected and should also not include any processed foods. After the elimination period, you reintroduce the food individually and pay close attention for any symptoms for about seventy-two hours. If you do not discern any reaction, consume the food again and wait another seventy-two hours. If there are no discernible symptoms, it may be okay to consume this food. But if you notice anything, even the worsening of reactions to other things, then it is in your best interest to avoid that food.

Although an elimination diet is a valid way to determine sensitivities and allergies to foods, it is many times very helpful to utilize laboratory testing. Conventional allergy testing primarily addresses an immunoglobulin known as IgE, which measures an immediate hypersensitivity reaction. Immediate hypersensitivity reactions, or Type I reactions, are usually determined with a scratch on or injection into the skin, and then watching for skin reactions like redness and swelling after a period of time. Today most allergists do not utilize this method for food testing; it is utilized more so for airborne allergens, and then treatment is initiated to change immune tolerance, thereby reducing a person's allergic symptoms. Reactions to food with this immunoglobulin can be very strong and even life-threatening. Immediate-hypersensitive foods are usually not treated with desensitization because of the serious level of reaction. Your only real tool is avoidance of the identified foods. Today, laboratories have improved the reliability of the RAST test, which can determine IgE reactions with blood samples. This is much safer than the skin testing and follow-up treatment.

There are other immunoglobulins to consider though, most notably IgG and IgA. A very common test for reactivity of IgG is called the ELISA test. This is commonly done to determine reaction to viruses and other foreign invaders in the body. IgG is part of the adaptive immune system and is actually more closely related to the food that you consume and digest because it is prominent in the bloodstream. In our clinic, we have found that IgG testing is an accurate and effective way to identify these IgG reactions. They are commonly called food sensitivities but are still immune responses. Referred to as delayed hypersensitivity, the IgG reactions may lead to symptoms of their own, but in my experience, I see more often that they increase the level of sensitivity of the entire immune system. I have many times identified IgG reactive foods and designed a food elimination strategy for those foods, only to see that people's reaction to airborne allergens is reduced or eliminated.

Your immune system is very complex; however, it can become quite sensitive if triggered chronically. If we can reduce the immune response level and frequency, many things that a person was sensitive to can be tolerated without symptoms. This can be accomplished by limiting foods that trigger an immune response. The body becomes overall less reactive and sensitive, helping to alleviate symptoms.

If you need or want to maintain a diet that is "gluten free," there are several grains and other choices for starch and flour that are considered acceptable. Corn, potato, yam, rice, tapioca, amaranth, arrowroot, millet, montina, lupin, quinoa, sorghum, taro, teff, and chia seed are acceptable substitutes, unless you determine that you have a reaction to one of these. In the United States, most people with gluten sensitivity usually avoid oats, while in Europe, gluten-sensitive people are encouraged to use oats. The major reason for this is that oats in United States are commonly processed with other grains and become contaminated with them. In Europe, the grains are processed separately. Generally oats without contamination are in fact safe to eat for many people, even with those with severe gluten sensitivity. The only caveat here is if someone reacts specifically to oats.

Flours produced from certain beans and nuts are also acceptable. Soybeans, many nuts, and other legumes can be used to produce a gluten-free product that tends to provide even more protein than many grains, along with better fiber content. Buckwheat, being different from actual wheat, can also be used, as well as flour from garbanzo beans (or gram flour—not to be confused with Graham flour, which is made from wheat).

Watch labels carefully, because gluten can be hidden as a food additive. You can find gluten in soup, gravy, soy sauce and other sauces, pasta, noodles, many meat products, and communion wafers. Gluten can be used as a stabilizing agent or thickener in products like ice cream and ketchup. Ingredients listed in any over-the-counter or prescription medications, and even vitamins, sometimes contain gluten. Cosmetics such as lipstick, lip balm, and lip gloss may contain gluten and should be investigated. Most products manufactured for Passover are gluten-free—except any foods that list matzo as an ingredient.

Before you stock up on gluten-free breads, keep in mind that bread is not really a naturally occurring food. It is a refined and processed grain product that has been altered to create flour. In the baking process, the flour is altered further for the browning reaction. This is the crust on your bread. The crust contains advanced glycation end products, which can damage your health. (See chapter 4.) Just because something claims that it is "gluten free" does not automatically mean that it is a healthy food to consume. Gluten-free foods can be just as processed and have just as much negative impact on our health. Sprouted grains, if less than ten days old, are more gluten free but cannot be guaranteed as being so. If you sprout seeds yourself, you can soak them to make them more digestible and retain some of the vitamins and minerals that would have been lost.

Dairy Products

Dairy products are responsible for many of the same problems. There are many people who cannot tolerate the milk of another animal. They also produce an immune response to the dairy proteins and sometimes fats. This can create a situation very similar to that with gluten. There are groups of people who tolerate raw dairy products and exhibit no reaction. For these people, consuming dairy can be a healthy habit. These same people cannot tolerate processed dairy products that have been pasteurized and homogenized, and usually contain antibiotics, growth factors, and other chemicals. It seems that the processing has actually altered the food enough to make it now unhealthy to consume.

Many scientists theorize that we are not designed to consume the milk of other animals. Others propose that it is not good for us to utilize milk for nutrition after weaning from our mothers. We are designed to consume human milk, perhaps not milk collected from other animals. We do know that some people have possibly evolved to use dairy and dairy products. Although there is not much evidence for the use of dairy during Paleolithic times, we do know that Northern European cultures and the Masai dating back to their indigenous roots indicate the use of dairy.

In terms of dairy products, it seems that there are different types of reactions to milk and its products. A lot of people don't produce the right enzyme to break down the sugar in milk called lactose. Inability to break down the sugar leads to digestive system symptoms, such as gas, bloating, and sometimes severe abdominal pain. Although it is not an immune response, it can create related symptoms. A large number of people do suffer an immune response to the milk solids commonly called casein, or caseinate. And fewer people experience an immune response even to the whey, or liquid portion of the milk after separation.

If you have an immune response to these proteins and fats, you will exhibit symptoms, and you are better off avoiding dairy. It is a good thing that there are many dairy substitutes. Milk substitutes are produced using rice, many nuts such as almonds or hazelnuts, coconut, soybean, and even sesame seeds. A good substitute for kids is oat milk or perhaps potato milk. Cheese and yogurt-like foods can also be made from these sources. In fact, presently there are many cheese-like foods that are actually dairy free. If you don't tolerate real dairy, try some of the imitation cheeses made from nuts. They actually melt like real cheese.

In a lot of cases, people may react to bovine products, or products from cows, but they seem to do quite well with dairy foods from goats or other animals. The specific-carbohydrate diet allows self-made goat yogurt, which you produce yourself from goat's milk. Also, as we stated earlier, a number of people can consume raw dairy without symptoms but do not tolerate pasteurization and other processing of dairy. It seems that pasteurization, homogenization, growth factors, and antibiotics also change the characteristics of the milk itself. Proteins and fats altered by processing become something different. If you suspect that dairy products are not good for you, I suggest that you at least eliminate dairy products from your diet to judge if you feel better. Elimination diets are an accurate way to determine if these foods are good for you. If you would rather, there are also laboratory tests that will indicate allergy or sensitivity to these foods. Just bear in mind that your body can react with any one or all of five groups of antibodies. Commonly the antibody classes IgE, IgG, or IgA are tested.

Other Genetically Modified Grains and Proteins

Let's not forget that there is also mounting evidence against the consumption of corn and corn products, as well as sorghum and soy. If these foods provided health benefits before, it seems that factory farming and genetic modification have aligned to reduce the value of these plants as food. There is even mounting scientific evidence that some of the chemicals present in many legumes can be detrimental to our health. Add to this the heavy use of pesticides and chemical fertilizers, which further detract from the value of these plants. The genetic modification of proteins is something that we need to be wary of, and this has already occurred to these particular types of plants.

Research tends to show conclusively that the foods valuable to health are vegetables, whole fruits, good sources of protein, and essential fats from nuts and seeds. Even today, in studies of hunter-gatherer groups who do not consume grains or dairy, modern diseases are not often found.

Many indigenous peoples like the Masai, Eskimos, and subarctic hunters even stay healthyconsuming only protein or fat.

It is quite possible to avoid grains, grain products, and dairy in your diet completely and thrive. In fact, if you're sensitive to it, your health may depend on it.

Chapter 4

Macronutrients

The Constituents of Food

We all need to obtain macronutrients on a regular basis. *Macronutrients* are the proteins, fats, and carbohydrates that you need to consume during your daily routine. Vitamins, minerals, and some plant chemicals are referred to as *micronutrients*, since they are only needed in a small amount. Nutrients are classified as either essential or non-essential. Essential nutrients are those that we have to consume, since they cannot easily be found or synthesized in the body. Non-essential nutrients are generally those that the body can synthesize or find a source for. Under certain circumstances, a nutrient may become "conditionally essential" when the body does not have enough available. For example, when you are stressed, you may use more B vitamins, even to a point of depleting your reserves. You need a higher amount than what you might normally intake. When you consume a diet that does not contain enough nutrients, your body will actually cannibalize itself to try to find enough of what it needs.

Are the proteins, fats, and carbohydrates that you consume good for you, or bad for you? Generally, if they are naturally occurring foods, your body will be able to use them appropriately, and you will create a state of good health. On the other hand, if these macronutrients are only naturally sourced, but then are processed and concentrated, you will likely create interference and dysfunction.

Protein

If you use animal products, did the animal live a natural life, consuming the foods it was designed to eat? Or did the animal grow up in a factory situation, forced to eat foods it would not naturally forage for, therefore altering that animal's state of health? In other words, do you eat healthy animals or sick animals?

If you don't consume animal products, you still need protein sources and the right balance of amino acids, as well as other nutrients. The same question becomes the issue. Were your foods raised in an industrialized situation, or did they naturally grow and therefore produce the nutrients that you really need? I have known many vegetarians claiming how healthy that lifestyle is, but they are far from healthy. In fact, the heaviest people I have worked with in our weight-loss program claimed to be vegetarian. What they really meant was that they did not eat animal products. The problem was that they consumed a great deal of processed food like breads, cereals, and pastas. Many consumed no vegetables at all, nor did they understand how to obtain the necessary nutrients.

When you consume proteins, they are generally digested into single amino acids or groups of amino acids. Your body will absorb these products from the protein and utilize them for many purposes in the body. It is very important to avoid proteins that have been altered. The body can always use natural proteins, but if we cook or process them too much, they become altered. Genetically modified foods contain modified proteins, which can cause altered function in the body. Protein deficiency can lead to symptoms such as fatigue, insulin resistance, hair loss, loss of muscle mass, low body temperature, hormonal irregularities, and neurotransmitter dysfunction. Severe protein deficiency can be fatal. Are your foods adulterated, full of chemicals, growth factors, or even genetically modified proteins?

The recommended daily allowance for protein is set at 0.36 grams of protein for every pound of your body weight. This is based on a concept called nitrogen balance. However, it has been found in studies that people who are more active, such as an athlete, will actually require as much as 2.5 grams of protein per pound of body weight. Generally, if you are physically active, a reasonable and sufficient protein intake works out to about 1 gram of protein per pound of body weight. This is especially true in endurance athletes, such as marathoners or triathletes, since they end up utilizing protein stores (muscle) as an energy source. If you perform activities that break down muscle, then it is imperative that you replace that protein. As far as percentage, current RDA recommendations are for protein to make up 15 percent of your diet. Again, there are very good studies in sports physiology showing a requirement for twice that. I tend to see most people do better if that percentage of protein approaches 30 percent.

There is a question of high-protein diets' affect on both liver and kidney function. It is true that these organs will need to work harder. It is not true that the higher protein intake, even above 30 percent, will in itself cause damage. In fact, the most dangerous situation for the liver results from high carbohydrate intake, which is converted to fat and creates a situation called fatty liver. Many people have utilized high-protein diets as well as high-fat diets to lose weight and even cure diseases without any ill effect. In any case, sufficient protein consumption can help to maintain and to increase muscle mass. The maintenance of muscle mass needs to be a daily priority, especially in the geriatric population.

We all need a proper balance of amino acids available. They are needed for immune system support as well as healthy cell growth. In fact, studies indicate that when we have sufficient amino acids available, we produce fewer abnormal cells. Our bone health is dependent upon proper protein intake. Too little protein and bones are weak and frail, while too much protein for an extended period can also produce an acid environment, leading to the thinning of bones.

Protein is an important component of every cell in the body. Your body uses protein to build and repair tissues and make enzymes, hormones, and other body chemicals. Protein is an important building block for bones, muscles, cartilage, skin, and even blood. Amino acids appear in a number of different forms, such as enzymes, keratin, elastin, collagen, hemoglobin, albumin, glycoproteins, antibodies, hormones, actin, and myosin. If you consume animals and animal products, you obtain a direct source of amino acids from the animals' complete protein. Whey protein from dairy, if processed properly, is actually a very good protein and has beneficial characteristics for the immune system and for the building of muscle tissue. Protein from fish tends to be easier to digest and is a good source of protein. Red meat tends to get a bad rap. If the animal ate its natural diet—for example, grass-fed beef or game meat—then the meat tends to be good for us. Industrialized, grain-fed feedlot meat can present many problems for health.

You can still get good protein if you don't consume animal products. Many vegetarians also consume certain animal products, such as fish, dairy, or eggs. Vegans who consume no animal products can still find many sources of protein. However, if you don't utilize animal products, you'll need to learn how to complement your proteins to get a complete balance of your amino acids. As long as you utilize vegetables, you can get some of your proteins, good fats, and carbohydrates. Consuming nuts and seeds also provides proteins and fats. Legumes such as beans are a source of protein; however, you have to realize that they also contain a lot of carbohydrates and may contain some natural chemicals that we don't want an excess of. If you plan to live vegetarian, just ensure that you are getting a good balance of your macronutrients and micronutrients. (A vegetarian diet can become deficient in vitamins such as B_6 and B_{12}, which are usually provided by consuming healthy animals.)

Proteins are made of chains of amino acids called peptides. Twenty different amino acids are present in the human body. Each amino acid can be used in different sequences connected together to provide the body with various proteins that it needs. Amino acid chains that are simple but long and straight tend to be used to build tissues, while proteins that are folded around themselves in a chain are called globular proteins, which are used for enzymes and other molecules inside the body. When you eat proteins, they must be properly digested so the body can absorb them and then actually reassemble them. A common problem is when people do not have enough stomach acid, or for some reason cannot properly break protein down, and therefore become protein deficient. The bottom line is to obtain sufficient protein.

Carbohydrates (Sugar)

Everybody just loves that sweet sensation. There are people that put sugar on, in, and around everything they eat. Many of us are not even aware of how much sugar we consume in beverages. Estimates on sugar consumption have gone from 2 to 4 pounds per person per year at the turn of the twentieth century up to—by some estimates—close to 200 pounds per person per year in the United States today. Conservative estimates place the consumption at somewhere around 143 pounds of sugar per person per year. That's a drastic change within a short span of time. The negative effects of concentrated and processed carbohydrates are catching up with us as well. Many of the diseases we are dealing with in our present society can be linked directly to sugar consumption and higher calorie intake overall. We have become a nation of carbohydrate junkies. This has not always been the case. It was not that long ago when people consumed whole foods that were more nutritionally sound and not concentrated into such a high dosage of empty calories.

However, we are told through marketing and the media that these food-like substances are wholesome and healthy. Manufacturers may make health claims based on a whole food, but they are selling that food after it is processed and very different from what it originally started from. Every day I work with patients in the clinic who believe they do not consume any sugar in their daily diet. It is not just a spoonful from the sugar bowl that we have to be concerned about. If you really start to pay attention and add up your calorie intake, especially from carbohydrates, most people will find that they are consuming a great deal of sugar. Flours or starchy foods are long chains of carbohydrates, and carbohydrates are sugars.

If you start adding up the consumption of bread, cereals, and convenience foods consumed, you will find a significant amount of sugar. And if you pay attention to all the sugar that you drink in sodas and juices, or add to food in the way of salad dressings and sauces, you will tend to find a very high carbohydrate intake. Do you know just how much sugar you can consume in a drink or juice? Most people would be hard pressed to simply eat several spoonfuls of sugar outright, yet many of the drinks in the way of sodas, fruit juices, and other drinks are loaded with numerous spoonfuls of sugar. Some of the drinks currently consumed by people contain as much as a quarter pound of sugar. The artificial sweeteners are no better, since studies have indicated that they stimulate cravings for even more sugar.

Many of us in the United States have moved to a diet almost completely composed of flour. These various flour-based foods contain no appreciable nutrients. If you consume these empty carbohydrates all day long, then you are creating a need for "triage." What this means is that you will be kept alive, but you will not be functioning at an optimal level. Practically speaking, this means more symptoms, less energy, and the production of diseases.

High Blood Sugar Levels Lead to Diabetes, Accelerated Aging, and Cancer

Researchers expect that by 2034 the number of people with diabetes will increase from 25 million to over 44 million, if nothing changes. Diabetes is currently such a common condition that people seem to ignore just how serious it really is. Diabetes is a very debilitating condition that creates very serious health complications. Since scientists and health professionals understand it to be more of a lifestyle disease, one has to wonder why it is so rampant. People do not "catch" or "have a genetically predetermined fate for" diabetes; it is primarily developed over time through poor lifestyle choices. Type I diabetes is a situation where little or no insulin is produced. Yet there are type I diabetics who are able to control their condition all or in part with lifestyle. They can at the very least reduce their reliance on insulin injections (exogenous insulin).

A large majority of type II diabetics develop diabetes because of poor lifestyle choices. The onset does not occur all in one day. It often takes years to develop diabetes, and if people change their lifestyle choices, they can reduce or eliminate the disease. Over time, as we consume a high-calorie diet, the body begins to become overwhelmed. The initial response is to try to keep up with higher blood sugar levels by producing more and more insulin. If the situation does not improve, eventually there is so much insulin present that the body will become insensitive to this very important hormone. Then, at some point, the body cannot produce enough insulin to control the level of sugar in the blood. This is how we create insulin insensitivity and diabetes.

There needs to be good control of the level of sugar in our blood. You actually have the most effective tools to do this in your hands. The answer is to control what you eat and drink. If you control your carbohydrate intake so that blood sugar levels don't rise too fast or too high, then you can retain your sensitivity to the insulin hormone. Most type II diabetics do produce sufficient insulin, but at some point when they cannot produce enough, they lose control. Ideally, between meals, the level of insulin is at a minimum, often close to zero. Then when blood sugar rises, insulin is produced and maintains a safe level of glucose. Usually, if a person watches the impact of sugar by eating low glycemic index foods (more on the glycemic index below), the system runs without a problem.

As insulin levels continue to rise, and even fasting levels remain higher, many people begin having a problem called reactive hypoglycemia. Most cases of hypoglycemia are really a secondary reaction to the overproduction of insulin. During this interim period of time, relatively high levels of insulin will actually drive blood sugar levels lower. With low blood sugar levels, it is hard to function because you have less energy, focus, and concentration. Many times your moods are affected, and this is a sign that the body is not getting enough in the way of energy. However, this is sort of the calm before the storm, and in these cases the low blood sugar levels are only preceding the onset of diabetes itself.

If you maintain a consistent and effective level of physical activity, then your body will transport and utilize the carbohydrates for energy. This mechanism of glucose transport will help keep things under control even independent of insulin. Exercise has the ability to transport sugar out of the blood without the presence of insulin, since exercise itself stimulates glucose (GLU T4) transporters. So, in a scenario of high carbohydrate intake and lessening physical activity, we literally lose control of the sugar content in the blood. When this control is impaired or lost, we are labeled as diabetics and treated with medications.

So if you make the right food choices and you are physically active, you can control the levels of sugar in your blood. If you simply monitor your fasting blood glucose levels, you have a good indicator of how you are doing. If your fasting glucose level is above 84 mg/dl in blood, then you enter the risk group for diabetes. If you do not maintain fasting control of your blood sugar, this is your early warning that there is a problem brewing. Researchers have demonstrated that a 6 percent increase in diabetes risk exists for every number above that 84 in your blood-sugar measurement.

It is unfortunate that many doctors will not even mention blood-sugar regulation until your levels are not maintained below 100 fasting, or the lab reference range. At this point they may say to you that you are pre-diabetic. Some doctors will wait until your number is above 140 fasting and then discuss with you the fact that you are diabetic. Now that you have reached this point, they can help you by offering drug therapy. I would prefer that you learn your risk for diabetes at a much earlier stage, where you have the ability to actually prevent it. Your health is not a wait-and-see situation; it will always be a better plan to maintain function and a physiological environment that does not allow disease. Think proactively and not reactively.

The current testing standard for diabetes is called hemoglobin A-1c. This is a measure spanning the life of your red blood cells. Now you have an estimate of your blood sugar levels over a period of about three months. If this percentage is above a certain reference range (I like to see it below 5 percent), then it is considered proof that you are diabetic. This test is actually indicating that your blood sugar levels have been high enough to react with the hemoglobin in your red blood cells. This percentage number will be higher or lower directly related to blood sugar.

As this percentage rises, the ability of the red blood cells to carry oxygen is impaired. This is a major problem, because if you can't carry and deliver oxygen to your tissues, then these tissues will die. Sugar becomes a danger to you when it is in excess and can react with proteins and fats in the body. So the excess sugar, above an acceptable level, is available to react and cause damage to you in a process called *glycation.*

When sugar reacts with, or glycates, body proteins and fats, it creates advanced glycation end products (or AGEs, for short). This glycation process hardens the arteries; damages critical muscles like the heart; breaks down the collagen structure of skin, bone, and other tissues; and can be a major source of free radicals. So if you let blood sugar levels remain elevated, then you are actually accelerating the aging process. It is currently understood that the physical changes we associate with aging are the result of free radical damage to the body. Free radicals are reactive molecules traveling through the body, destabilizing tissues by oxidizing them. These "free radicals," or reactive molecules, steal electrons from molecules and tissues and cause damage to you. Most people tend to notice the damage the most when collagen is affected. When collagen is damaged by oxidation, this leaves you with wrinkles, thin and fragile skin, osteoporotic bones without good structure, and a list of changes in your appearance and your health. Symptoms begin and eventually diseases are created, because of the damage to your own anatomy.

Normally, the largest source of free radicals comes from every breath that you take. Oxygen, when used in the body, creates reactive oxygen species (free radicals) that have a purpose, but if not kept under control, they can also cause physical damage. However, in people that consume excess sugar, the major source of free radicals are these advanced glycation end products. The more free radicals that are present, the more damage that will occur.

Why would the body create something that does damage? While there is a purpose for free radicals, your body also has a way to deal with them. Free radicals are used in the body as a defense mechanism and also to run certain necessary reactions. But as I stated, you have a way to control these and other free radicals. These control molecules are referred to as antioxidants. You've probably heard this term frequently and very likely have taken some product, food, or supplement that promised to have high antioxidant activity. Some sources of antioxidants, especially antioxidant-containing foods, in many cases actually stimulate our own production of these important molecules.

Generally your best and most abundant source of effective antioxidants are those that you produce yourself inside your body. When you exercise, you will generate lots of free radicals. At the same time, though, you will produce an overabundance of antioxidants—molecules like glutathione, super oxide dismutase, and others produced by your body for your body. You actually produce many more antioxidants than you will need for the free radicals produced during exercise. Therefore, you can experience a net gain of antioxidants.

If you consume real foods, you also consume antioxidants, or more commonly you consume plant chemicals formed under stress that stimulate your body to produce more of its own antioxidants in response. In either case, real, natural, whole food can protect you, offering substances that trigger the body to produce more antioxidants, and some foods even contain and are a supply of actual antioxidants. You can also take supplements such as alpha-lipoic acid, glutathione in an absorbable form, coenzyme Q10, and other molecules that have antioxidant capability to aid your body in the control of these free radicals.

In past years, sugar was actually advertised as a healthy substance that would provide energy and health, so people were encouraged to use more.

But we now have to consider the fact that more sugar can overwhelm the body, leading to diabetes, heart disease, hypertension, high cholesterol, osteoarthritis, osteoporosis, cancer, and aging. To some extent, it probably plays a part in the mechanism of every disease. Fructose, also known as fruit sugar, was touted as a more healthy option until we understood the mechanisms of carbohydrates more accurately.

Table sugar, or sucrose, consumed in excess is known to cause health problems. Sucrose will cause dysfunction in its concentrated form, but it is made up of one part glucose and one part fructose. The human body detects glucose and bases its response on sugar concentration. Therefore, at least sucrose is perceived and detected by the body when it enters. This means that the body can ready a response, including the release of insulin to keep the sugar level under control. Again, when not overwhelmed, the system works fine.

Today the primary source of sugar has become fructose, in the form of high-fructose corn syrup. This is also called fruit sugar, or corn sugar. Fruit sugar, or fructose, in small amounts consumed from whole fruit is not really a problem. Most fruit contains fiber, and during the digestive process, the digestion of fruit and the absorption of fructose is slowed. If we process and concentrate fructose, and then consume it in large amounts, fructose is actually more dangerous than other types. In the past, fructose was looked at as the "safe sugar," since fructose did not stimulate a strong insulin response. However, it turns out that the fructose acts more like a ninja, sneaking into the body and causing damage before you know it is there.

Since corn is heavily subsidized, its byproducts are relatively inexpensive for industrial food producers to purchase. This is one of the reasons that it's used so extensively. Although the marketing is aimed at convincing you that sugar is sugar, if you study the mechanisms of sugar, you will see this is not the case. Your available food is heavily influenced by politics and farm subsidies, not by nutritional science.

As medical science continues to advance, better and better methods are being found to detect health problems. Positron emission tomography scans are a unique type of imaging test that helps doctors see how the organs and tissues inside your body are actually functioning. The test involves injecting a very small dose of a radioactive chemical, called a radiotracer, into the vein of your arm. The tracer travels through the body and is absorbed by the organs and tissues being studied. This machine detects and records the energy given off by the tracer substance and, with the aid of a computer, this energy is converted into three-dimensional pictures. A physician can then look at cross-sectional images of the body organ from any angle in order to detect any functional problems.

One of the most effective ways now available to detect and to monitor the extent of cancer in the body is the PET scan. This is been a major advancement for doctors when they need to identify cancer's location. A PET scan can measure such vital functions as blood flow, oxygen use, and glucose metabolism, which helps doctors distinguish abnormal from normal functioning organs and tissues. The scan can also be used to evaluate the effectiveness of a patient's treatment plan, allowing the course of care to be adjusted if necessary.

Glucose, or sugar, is radioactively tagged in a solution, which is then injected into the body. The scan demonstrates exactly where the sugar travels to in your body. Let's think about this for a moment: if you follow where sugar goes in the human body, you will find that it goes to metabolically active tissues: some goes to the brain, some to the gonads, but a large amount straight to any cancer cells. Cancer cells need sugar and will do everything they can to take all they can get. Some of the most promising and effective treatments for cancer include starving cancer cells by reducing sugar. Create a state of ketosis, and cancer cells die. Ketones are byproducts of fat breakdown. Cancer cells can't run on ketones, but your body is actually designed to. You can literally starve the cancer and drive it into remission while your body receives a better fuel from fats.

To the contrary, if you provide sugar in abundance, you create the environment for cancer to flourish. This means even if you have not developed cancer yet, you are giving cancer cells their best chance if you overconsume sugar. Oncologists are currently realizing that if they don't monitor sugar levels and sugar intake, they may prolong treatment and reduce its effectiveness. Many of the current cancer drugs can lose as much as 90 percent of their effectiveness when sugar is consumed.

When patients undergo chemotherapy, radiotherapy, or cancer-debulking surgery, they can end up in a catabolic or wasted state, becoming very frail and underweight. The first thing we want to do for these people is feed them calories so that they will put on more weight. We have to be very careful here, though; because if we just feed these people cakes and candies and other forms of sugar, we may just preferentially strengthen the cancer that we were trying to weaken. This may prolong the time required for cancer therapy and even render the therapy ineffective.

Another example of the effect of sugar on your body comes from studies done on your white cells and other immune system cells. When these cells are being studied and are active, it has been observed that the administration of sugar will slow down and even stop them from working altogether. It has also been demonstrated that people with higher blood sugar levels have less effective immune cells. So, if you consume too much sugar without adequate control, then your immune system will be impaired and even become unresponsive.

Other studies demonstrate that in cases of high blood sugar, we create a situation that is termed *metabolic syndrome,* or syndrome X. The most important risk factors for this are extra weight around the middle and insulin resistance. If you have three or more of the following signs, you have metabolic syndrome.

- Blood pressure 130/85 mm/hg or higher
- Fasting blood sugar 100 mg/dL or higher
- A man with a waist measuring 40 inches or more, or a woman 35 inches or more
- Low HDL cholesterol: a man under 40 mg/dl or a woman under 50 mg/dL
- Triglycerides 150 mg/dL or more, new level below 100

As blood sugar levels go higher, arterial stiffness, or hardening of the arteries, happens at a very advanced rate compared to normal. This is a mechanism whereby increased sugar intake produces hypertension, stroke, and heart disease. Numerous studies have demonstrated that the risk or incidence of cancer climbs linearly with the increase in fasting glucose levels. Uncontrolled sugar definitely leads to cancer and diseases of all kinds.

When tissue samples of skin or collagen are studied, you can actually see a difference in tissue integrity related directly to blood sugar levels. Even the Centers for Disease Control and the American Medical Association have recognized studies linking high-fructose corn syrup with obesity, higher incidence of diabetes, and many other conditions.

The Toxicity of Sugar

Because sugar is capable of being a toxic substance to the body, an extremely important strategy is to control blood glucose levels within a tight range. For example, sugar places unnecessary stress on the system, and that means a rise of adrenaline and other stress hormones like cortisol. Now you're looking at sleep problems, weight problems, and even creating a situation of hyperactivity, anxiety, difficulty concentrating, and moodiness in adults, or crankiness in children. High sugar intake also can cause high triglycerides and a decrease in HDL or good cholesterol; this puts you at risk for heart and vascular disease. Also, there tends to be a rise in total cholesterol and the LDL cholesterol.

There is a loss of tissue elasticity and function. You now know that cancer is fed by sugar and has been directly connected with development of cancer of the breast, ovaries, prostate, rectum, pancreas, biliary tract, lung, gallbladder, and stomach.

As they begin to overuse sugar, people often develop reactive hypoglycemia as the body tries to produce enough insulin to control the runaway sugar. In the beginning, the pancreas puts out too much because of the alarm response, and your blood sugar levels tend to be driven too low. But eventually the body becomes less sensitive to the insulin, and the pancreas cannot produce enough.

Sugar can weaken eyesight because of the damage done to the small capillaries and other structures of the eye. You will have problems in your gastrointestinal tract, including higher acid levels outside of the stomach, indigestion, and malabsorption, and there is a definite connection between sugar and Crohn's disease, ulcerative colitis, and other inflammatory bowel disorders.

Sugar causes premature aging. It is related to alcoholism, tooth decay, gum disease, and a Pandora's box of disease. It produces obesity, inflammation, autoimmune disease and is grain fed responsible for creating an environment where pathogens can flourish. One of the most common problems with high sugar is an overgrowth of candida albicans, or what's commonly called a yeast infection.

There are studies tying sugar intake to gallstones, appendicitis, hemorrhoids, varicose veins, and osteoporosis. Oral contraceptive users have a much higher incidence of diabetes and loss of blood sugar control. Sugar tends to lower vitamin E levels and increases systolic blood pressure. It can cause drowsiness, sleep apnea, and narcolepsy. It interferes with the absorption of essential proteins and increases food allergies. It sets up a toxic environment, such as toxemia during pregnancy.

It contributes to eczema in children, atherosclerosis and cardiovascular disease in adults, and it's been shown to impair the structure and repair of your DNA. It can change the structure of a protein and permanently alter the way the proteins act in your body. Hormones cannot work normally and are unable to reach the receptors.

Sugar causes cataracts and nearsightedness. It is linked to emphysema. It can impair enzyme function. There is a higher incidence of Parkinson's disease and Alzheimer's. Sugar will increase the size of your liver by increasing the production of triglycerides and fat that can deposit in liver cells. Sugar tends to increase the kidney size, produce kidney stones, and cause kidney dysfunction. It can damage your pancreas. It can increase fluid retention and constipation. It compromises circulation in tendons, muscles, and other tissues. It can produce headaches, reduce learning capacity, cause learning disorders, and it can change the actual brain waves.

Sugar leads to depression, even though it is thought of as the short-term fix for serotonin levels. Sugar increases your risk for gout. Sugar creates hormone imbalances, increasing estrogen in men, exacerbating PMS in women, and decreasing growth hormone in both. Sugar leads to dizziness and peripheral vascular disease, increases platelet adhesion, and is being linked to premature infants and smaller for gestational age infants. IVs of sugar have been known to cut off oxygen to the brain. Sugar increases the risk of polio, increases the risk of epileptic seizures, and it causes higher blood pressure. Sugar can induce cell death.

The Glycemic Index

The secret to an optimally functioning body is to consume the fewest calories necessary while receiving the most nutrients possible. If you depend on processed food-like substances that are essentially flour and sugar throughout the entire day, you're consuming lost of calories, but hardly any nutrients. A number of recent studies are pointing to higher concentrated calorie intake as the cause of mental and physical disorders. Notably, Alzheimer's disease and dementia have been tied to this type of high-calorie diet.

As a culture, few of us understand anymore what real food is. So even if you make the decision to eat real food, you may still struggle with knowing exactly what to eat in the place of the processed convenience foods that you are used to. We need a better way to judge our foods. One tool that I think works very well is to learn the *glycemic index* of foods. Practically every food has been indexed, both real foods and processed foods. Tables and algorithms can be found on the Internet, in books, and even in software. The glycemic index is a measurement of the impact of the food on your blood sugar levels. If you consume lower glycemic index foods, you will have less impact.

High glycemic index foods, such as sugar, white flour, white rice, processed grains, other junk foods, and many tropical and dried fruits, will quickly raise blood sugar to higher levels faster and stimulate more insulin production, starting a cycle that, as explained above, can lead to diabetes and other health problems.

Less impact on blood sugar levels and on insulin production means less impact on your health. Low glycemic index foods promote weight loss, while preserving lean muscle mass and increasing your metabolic rate. Low glycemic index foods allow your body to produce a steady stream of energy. If you pay attention to the glycemic index, you can avoid insulin resistance, as well as the physical damage done by excess sugar and insulin in the blood.

As the glycemic index indicates, there are also beneficial carbohydrates. Fiber intake is a very important carbohydrate, or sugar. It is not digestible by the human body in many cases. Fiber cleans out the digestive tract. In fact, the incidence of diverticulosis and diverticulitis goes to zero with enough fiber intake. Fiber also is able to absorb toxins, excess sugars, and fats and allows your body to eliminate them. The most important job for fiber is to feed your own probiotics. These are the organisms that live in the digestive tract. These organisms provide some vitamins like vitamin K, they provide enzymes so you can more effectively digest food, and they actually protect the digestive tract. Even more importantly, the probiotics teach your immune system what to attack and what to tolerate. This is a very important task.

If probiotics are not present, then your immune system can easily start mistaking your tissue for something that should be dealt with. The immune cells work by recognizing pathogens' associated molecular patterns (PAMPs). Without the help of your friendly organisms, your immune system may begin to attack you. This is called autoimmune disease, and there is a lot of research demonstrating the connection between probiotics and these diseases. Autoimmunity looks different depending on which tissue is attacked. Rheumatoid arthritis, Hashimoto's thyroiditis, systemic lupus, Sjogren's, and many other diseases are autoimmune processes. Interestingly, when people have one, they tend to develop others. Autoimmunity is now more recognized as an overall condition of the body. Probiotics are possibly a very effective treatment to restore your tolerance to you.

If you don't have control of sugar, then you are suppressing your immune system and impairing your own defense against infectious disease. You require certain nutrients, such as chromium and copper and B vitamins, to process the excess sugar, and you may impair absorption of other nutrients. The sugars you're eating may not contain enough nutrients, and they may deplete the nutrients that you do have.

As the glycemic index climbs over 100, you are looking at almost entirely processed foods. Cakes, candies, cookies, and other snacks have a higher glycemic index because their sugar is so readily available and will raise blood glucose levels immediately. Real food commonly has a lower glycemic index and the advantage of not shocking the body and raising blood sugar levels.

An even more accurate number than the glycemic index is called the *glycemic load*. This is an adjusted glycemic index taking into account each food's sugar content for the amount consumed. The glycemic index is not a perfect measure, but it is an easy way to make a fairly accurate judgment of food. There are tables to be found for this too. I suggest that you keep the glycemic index number somewhere around 55. The goal is to control for radicals, not necessarily eliminate them. But you don't want your free radicals to be primarily in the form of advanced glycation end products.

Once you master glycemic index, then investigate the glycemic load. The final step is to consider the glycemic complexing of your entire meal. It requires a little math, but it allows for the fact that higher glycemic indexes are mediated by lower ones considering the total foods consumed in a meal.

If you need an even easier system to judge your foods, then consider the rule of avoiding white foods. If the food has no color naturally, it is likely primarily a starch or sugar.

I fully understand, though, that we do live in the modern world. I am not trying to lead you to a lifestyle where you can never enjoy and celebrate. By all means, when there are festivals, holidays, birthdays, or any other reasons to celebrate, it is absolutely okay to indulge. Bread, in fact, was a festival food. There are even known advantages to spiking your blood sugar and insulin for the purpose of changing body structure and building muscle tissue. Some substances when taken for a short time can have benefit; however, they will hurt you if taken for a longer period of time. Therefore, it is sometimes appropriate to load carbohydrates with the goal of raising blood sugar, glycogen levels, and insulin levels. If this is done correctly, the body will compensate in ways that help adaptation and physical performance. For example, a bodybuilder might eat a high-carbohydrate meal in order to get a rise in insulin, which will enhance the transport of amino acids and synthesis of muscle. There are many occasions where making a change in your exercise routine periodically will move you forward. However, it is not appropriate to shock your body every day. I suggest that you can enjoy yourself perhaps once a week and still maintain very good health.

Fats

For many years, fat in the diet was blamed for everyone's weight and health problems. However, now we know that some fats are good and that they are necessary for your health and survival. It turns out to be a real mistake to avoid the intake of good fat. There are fats that will promote and sustain healthy function, and certain other types of fats that are bad and will destroy your health. As you might have guessed, the naturally occurring fats, which we get in natural foods and sometimes through supplements, are the beneficial ones. If fats are altered from their natural configuration by processing, the body may try to use them; however, human physiological function suffers. This means that your health suffers.

Good fats occur naturally in nuts, seeds, algae, plants, and to some extent in other animals that we eat. This is only true if that animal lived consuming its natural diet. Fats that are not good for us are the ones that have been altered through the application of heat, light, pressure, or various chemical reactions. These "altered" fats will lead to altered physiological function. Fats are a structural component of cells and molecules that function in the human body and keep it healthy. Most of them occur in a molecular formation described as cis, although some natural fats do occur in a trans molecular formation as well. In the cis form, a molecule—though it may be a long string of atoms—has both ends pointing in the same direction. If the molecule has a trans structure of the molecule, one end is oriented in one direction and the other in a different or opposite direction. This difference in the form of the molecule changes its shape and its characteristics.

Since fats are used to build the human cells' plasma membrane, hormones, neurotransmitters, and immune-modulating molecules, the structure of the fat makes a difference. When the fat molecule is altered or different from the naturally occurring molecule, it also changes the characteristics of anything the fat is to be used for. Processed fats, when taken into the body, are still utilized, but since their molecular structure is changed, the characteristics of whatever the fat is being used for are also changed. This is why many trans fats are considered dangerous to your health and why recent laws require them to be listed on labels. Many heart and circulation problems are traced back to the type of fat consumed.

Food manufacturers alter fats to intentionally change their characteristics when outside of the body. For example, as a substitute for butter, oils are processed into margarine using heat and pressure to alter their structure. The most common molecular alteration is to change a fat from the cis formation to the trans formation. These are then what are commonly referred to as trans fats. The molecule has literally been twisted, and it loses certain characteristics, like flexibility. When you consume these altered fats, and they are put in the place of the natural fats, you actually alter both structure and function.

These new properties of the fat are used to hold baked goods together so they don't crumble apart. Fats are altered so that instead of having liquid properties, they act more like a solid. Also, when you alter fats they won't go bad (rancid) and have a long shelf life. A fat "spoils" in its' reaction to light and air, but this reactivity allows your body to use the fat effectively. To change these same characteristics, changes the fats value for health. When you heat the fat, the food changes, or cooks. When fats and sugars undergo the browning effect of cooking, you have changed the sugar or fat. The more you change the food from its natural state, the more there will be consequences affecting your health and wellness.

Fats consumed in their natural state are generally very flexible and fluid like. Fats are an efficient way to store energy, containing over twice as much potential caloric energy as proteins or carbohydrates (e.g., nine calories per gram of fat versus four calories per gram of either carbohydrate or protein). Your body converts excess carbohydrates and stores them with dietary fats to be used later for energy. Fats are used in the construction of your cells. Human cells are very active; there is a lot going on at the surface of the cell. Animal cells have a plasma cell membrane that contains and isolates the organelles and other contents of the cell. Plant cells, on the other hand, have an actual cell wall. The human plasma membrane of the cell is very fluid and dynamic, having a lot of flexibility. The plasma membrane has been referred to as the brain of the cell. There are many decisions to be made at this level, and so much going on, that it is almost like the cell itself is thinking and reacting for you.

This flexible and fluid like plasma membrane contains receptors for many hormones, antibodies, and kinases (molecules that help us communicate in the body), and carries on many essential and critical functions. It acts as a barrier for the cell, but it also allows diffusion of certain molecules and has the ability to pump or transfer things into or out of the cell. Nutrients must be selectively allowed into the cell. Waste products are gathered and carried out of the cell. Osmotic pressure and fluid balance are extremely critical functions at the plasma membrane. You can actually determine the health of the cell by measuring the fluid content inside the cell and outside the cell.

The human cell membrane is made up of a phospholipid (fat) double layer. It is constructed from natural fats. As you consume more altered or trans fats, then the body will try to use the trans fats in constructing the plasma cell membrane. When these trans fats are utilized, the cell membrane becomes more stiff and almost impenetrable. This means the plasma membrane cannot function in the same fashion as before. To illustrate this, I want you to visualize a child's Lego block collection used for construction. If the plastic blocks are formed correctly and uniformly, you can build an intricate structure that holds together well, has good form, and functions as it is designed to. If you were to heat the plastic blocks so that they were soft enough, and then twist several blocks a half turn and let them cool, it would be much more difficult to build anything useful.

If you build a cell's outside membrane with trans fats, instead of being very fluid, flexible, and selectively porous, the cell membrane will stiffen, and all activity around and inside the cell will be affected. As I mentioned, cell membranes contain receptors for hormones, immune-modulating chemicals, and even antibodies. There are specific receptors for all the major hormones in your body, and they are found on most cell surfaces. These receptors are made of protein and have a glove like configuration, selectively allowing only certain hormones to enter and cause an effect, or hormone response. If we remember that hormones are major messengers in the body that need receptors to deliver their message, the effects of interference to this communication becomes more apparent.

These receptors at the surface are known to have mobility, and they do move out at certain times in anticipation of certain hormones and the expected effects. The hormone receptors then turn away at certain times, just like a baseball player who folds his glove when he does not expect to catch a baseball. For example, during the female menstrual cycle, at certain times of the month, the estrogen receptor will move out and open wider to accept estrogen. At other times during the month, the receptor is less accessible to estrogen, having moved to a different direction. A logical solution for this is often to add more hormones when symptoms of hormone deficiency appear. This will actually make things worse, since we are dealing with the problem of receptors, not inadequate hormones. A more appropriate solution is to correct the ability of the receptors to operate normally so they are sensitive to the hormone.

You may actually perceive a hormone deficiency, then, when the actual problem truly lies in the availability of hormone receptors. If you stiffen up the cell membrane, then antibodies and other receptors are unable to move or function in their normal manner. When the plasma membrane loses flexibility, it can also transmit an undulation, or a wave along its surface, which is destructive. If the membrane remains very fluid, a disturbance in the membrane will be localized. When the membrane is less flexible, then waves are transmitted further, gain velocity, and are more powerful. Scientist call this the "tsunami effect," and it can actually destroy the cell surface, much like a tsunami can destroy a city. There are many more examples where changing the characteristics of the cell membrane will cause imbalances, dysfunction, or disease.

Fats provide the raw materials to build your brain and your nervous system. It is interesting to note that when a woman becomes pregnant, her brain will literally shrink in size to meet the needs of the fetus. If her nutritional intake of certain fats is limited, her brain will shrink even more. The developing fetus will get what it needs to the detriment of the mother. The baby literally steals fats from the mother's body and brain during the formation of its own brain. It is actually very accurate to assume that a mother loses her mind when she becomes pregnant. The mother's brain will also rebuild back to normal size, if there is adequate nutrition after delivery of the child.

If essential fats are not available for the brain and nervous system, these structures cannot work as well as they should. We need DHA to build the structure of our brains and nervous system, and we need EPA for the proper function of both. Lacking essential fats will limit your ability to learn information or skills and even to concentrate or remember. It is now accepted that learning is in part a process of the myelination of nerves as they are repeatedly used. Myelin is a protective coating around the nerve, almost like the insulation on electrical wires. But the myelin also facilitates the electrical signal, allowing it to go faster and be delivered more efficiently. Your thoughts, actions, and other nerve impulses literally travel better over a myelinated neural network. Scientists have found that when you are learning, you actually further develop that part of the neural network that is being used. You will form a much better myelin sheath around nerves that you're using, and the nerves will grow larger and more resilient. That is, if you have the raw materials, or essential fats, available.

If we use a certain part of our neural network, those particular nerves being utilized will increase in size, have better trophic flow (or nutrient delivery), and develop a better myelin sheath. When we don't use certain nerves, they begin to lose the myelin coating and even go through a process of pruning and destruction. Understand that the human body, your body, is constantly undergoing change in response to how you use it. You are either facilitating a process of regenerating your body or allowing its degeneration. Either response is directly reflective of your lifestyle. If the proper nutrients are not available, then our adaptive processes may not be able to continue in the right way.

Fats are necessary for the absorption of certain important nutrients. One of the biggest problems with a low-fat diet is that you will become deficient in certain nutritional molecules. Vitamin A, vitamin D, vitamin E, vitamin K, coenzyme Q10, and many other nutrients will not be absorbed and utilized in the absence of adequate fat intake. Essential fats are necessary for the body, and we must be careful to include them in our diet every day. Even the modern low-fat diets are designed so that you will receive the good fats. If you don't intake good fats or are not able to process them correctly, you tend to create a situation of inflammation in the body. You especially need EPA to help control your immune response. Virtually any disease process in the body stems from inflammation.

It is very common today for people to over consume saturated fats and become deficient in those that are unsaturated. Many years ago, people consumed a ratio close to 1:1. They were consuming as much unsaturated fat as they were saturated fats. In our modern culture, we tend to take in enough saturated fat, but we are really missing unsaturated fats. Some people consume a saturated to unsaturated ratio of about 20:1. This is often because they also consume animals whose fat ratios are way out of balance and utilize corn oil and high omega 6 sources. For example, the meat of grain-fed industrially produced cattle ends up containing mostly saturated fats, whereas the meat of grass-fed cattle will contain a much higher ratio of unsaturated fats. Wild fish, or in some cases fish that are supplemented with unsaturated fats, become a good source of essential fats basically because of their diet.

Fats are components in the actual structure of hormones. We all know that we need hormones, in their proper physiological levels and ratios, for the body itself to function correctly. Hormones facilitate communication throughout the body. They are part of the regeneration, adaptation, and the maintenance of the body itself, and of your health. Some hormones offer neural protection, keeping your nervous system functioning and safe. Hormones are important in the prevention and control of cancer, and not a cause for cancer. In our clinic, the goal is to primarily utilize bio-identical hormones, or hormone molecules that have the same structure as the hormones that your body produces.

For example, estrogen in the blood is dependent on the amount of fat in the human body. Once the fat percentage of a female's normal body weight drops below 15 percent, menstruation is likely to stop temporarily. Females who are doing intense physical training, adolescents with anorexia, and overly lean teenagers are likely to have delayed menstruation. At the other extreme, as people gain weight their estrogen levels will go higher, since the fat cells themselves are classed as endocrine organs and, among other things, can produce estrogen.

Ideally, we strive to bring the levels of hormones to within the range normally experienced physiologically. In the absence of certain fats, the human body lacks the raw materials to even produce the hormones that you need. Hormone levels are ever-changing in response to your lifestyle and in response to each other. When you produce hormones, they do their required jobs, and then you metabolize them into other molecules and eventually even eliminate them from your body. Your health is dependent on this entire mechanism taking place safely to the finish. When you're not using natural hormones that the body recognizes, then you tend to disrupt this normally safe mechanism. In studies that point to the dangers of hormone replacement, they are most likely studies on hormones that have a different configuration.

Note that chemical pesticides and other pollutants, also called persistent organic pollutants, will tend to be stored in the body fat. The higher the fat content of the food, the more pesticides and pollutants it may contain. Be careful of high-fat foods that are not organic.

The current buzz about cholesterol, which is a fat, and heart disease is being redirected. It turns out that medical science has uncovered what is behind heart and vascular problems. It actually comes down to inflammation, oxidative stress, and the body's own immune response. Modern doctors can no longer base their decisions on a total cholesterol number. It is not even a good indicator of your risk, and the number gives no information on how to proceed with treatment. Cholesterol-lowering drugs are not for everyone, and their real value is to check the inflammatory process. Most of the evidence for their use is for treatment of second events or people who've already had a heart attack. As prevention, their success is limited.

Statins do lower cholesterol, but it is their effect on more accurate risk factors that should be considered. Cholesterol drugs also have serious side effects and should only be used when you have more information than the total cholesterol. In many cases, there are more effective and safer ways to get these same effects. By using more accurate biomarkers that can be measured in the blood, we can get a much better picture of what that patient's situation is. Sometimes a statin drug, fibrate, or other medication may be the best approach. However, the best treatment is to design a comprehensive and individualized strategy based upon a more complete assessment. Many of the people who visit our clinic do not want to use statins or other medications. We will order more accurately designed laboratory assessments and, based on those results, implement a plan of treatment, not just a pill.

Before I would consider using any of these drugs on a patient, I would want to know if they are at risk, and I would want to know the reasons why they are risk. Today there are several tests that can demonstrate actual risk factors and tell me if I should even utilize medication. In every case, it will be a multifactorial approach, and the first thing I will address is the patient's lifestyle. If testing indicates that there is vascular dysfunction in your body, the best resource that you have is proper food and exercise. Lifestyle will literally change the markers of risk. The next step is to see what nutrients can be used as a nutraceutical to influence each person's body to work better and eventually change these biomarkers of risk. The final step is to determine if medication is necessary or helpful in the short term. This way I can put the patient on their path towards health instead of simply taking control.

I bring this up since I am seeing many patients who I believe are overmedicated. Using drugs to reduce cholesterol to the lowest number possible creates more problems than it solves. In many cases, cholesterol is reduced to such a low level that there is not enough for the body, and the patient is in a hormone-deficient state. Cholesterol is a safe and necessary fat that the body produces as a hormone source and as a response to stress. If cholesterol is too low, we cannot produce good physiological levels of hormones. Cholesterol is only dangerous when it becomes oxidized, glycated, or otherwise altered. More importantly, we need to know the cholesterol particle size and overall number. Now I have a better idea what is actually going on. If we uncover a problem, eventually the answer is to keep your cholesterol safe and to prevent the process of inflammation. Generally our bodies produce the majority of cholesterol, although some people can absorb it. It is true that if you lower total cholesterol, you have less cholesterol that could be altered and become dangerous. This may sound logical on the surface; however, we have to consider the overall and long-term effects.

If there is reason for concern about heart disease, cholesterol, or the fact that in your family history there is incidence of vascular disease, make sure you get the right laboratory testing. At the very least, certain markers of inflammation and metabolism should be assessed. C-reactive protein, homocysteine, and Lp(a) are becoming more mainstream. I recommend that you request a full lipid sub-fraction panel. There are many laboratories offering these assessments.[3] Presently in our clinic we are having very good success with the panel of laboratory tests provided by Boston Heart Labs. By doing a more accurate assessment, we can actually see more of what is going on. We can answer questions such as: Is your LDL cholesterol safe? Is your HDL cholesterol working? Do you have inflammation of the vascular endothelium? Do you have the added risk of blood sugar dysregulation?—and much more. With more accurate information, we can implement a much more effective strategy.

Good fats are necessary to have beautiful, healthy skin. There are so many products out there used to treat the skin. All these topical applications of nutrients, steroids, creams, lotions, and other substances can help the skin to heal. It is true that you can deliver nutrients and other good things right through the skin. In my opinion, the best answer is to create healthy skin from the inside, because in most cases the skin is reflecting what is going on internally. If your body has the correct dietary nutrients, especially good dietary fats, you will produce the healthy skin everyone is searching for. Of course, some things coming in contact with the skin will cause a reaction, and this may have to be dealt with through medication to mediate the immune response. However, the majority of skin conditions come from some imbalance within the body. It can be as simple as correcting a nutritional deficiency or blood sugar issues, or it may be the presence of an autoimmune process that can be mediated.

Fat forms a protective cushion for your internal organs. You do need a certain amount of fat for various purposes beyond the storage of energy. One of the uses in the body for fat is as a protective cushion for your organs and other body structures. However, if too much fat accumulates, this cushion becomes a source of danger. Fat cells are now classified as endocrine organs themselves. They actually produce hormones like estrogen, adiponectin, leptin, and several cytokines, which are inflammatory promoters. As you accumulate more fat, you actually become more inflamed inside. This is especially true locally where there is a concentration of fat. When too

3 Just to name a few: the Boston Heart Lab panel, the Berkeley test, the Cleveland HeartLab panel, the Vertical Auto Profile (VAP), the Lipoprotein Particle Profile (LPP), and the cardiovascular panel from Metametrix labs.

much fat accumulates near an internal organ, that organ can suffer from the excess of inflammatory response and even sustain permanent damage. Excess fat will accumulate within the cells of an organ and impair the function of that organ. Research is noting fat accumulation in liver cells, bone cells, muscle cells (this is especially alarming when it is the muscle of the heart or liver), and other areas where it does not belong.

The more dangerous deposition of fat is called visceral adipose tissue. When you accumulate fat around your major organs, it creates what is referred to as the "apple" shape. It is safer, and more common in women, to have a "pear" shape. The pear-shaped body is actually less prone to disease because the fat has accumulated more around the hips. In the apple shape, there is a lot of fat right around the internal organs producing inflammatory chemicals. There is a much higher incidence of cardiovascular disease with this type of body shape, as well as organ dysfunction. Fats are pleasurable to consume, adding texture and taste to food. If our food does not contain any fat, it loses its consistency and taste, so people tend to use more sugar. Just like your mind will crave sugar, your mind is also seeking out good fats. Fat-free foods tend to be pretty bland, even tasteless.

Fats have different characteristics depending on the degree of saturation. Fats consist of a carbon chain, often with a carboxyl group at the end. When hydrogens are attached to every carbon, and there are no open double bonds, then the fat is a "saturated" fat. There are monounsaturated fats with one area open, and there are polyunsaturated fats. Depending on how many open or "unbound" carbons there are in the chain, the characteristics of the fat will be different. A saturated fat will tend to be solid at room temperature and not quite as flexible as one that is unsaturated. Monounsaturated fats, with a single unbound site, have a different configuration and are slightly more flexible then saturated.

Polyunsaturated fats have more than one unbound site, and because of this are even more flexible and reactive. When sites are unbound, the fat molecule is also more chemically reactive to other molecules and structures. Saturated fats are commonly found in animal products but are also found naturally in some plants. A healthy saturated fat is found as a medium-chain triglyceride (MCT) in coconuts. Monounsaturated fats are commonly consumed from foods like olive oil. Polyunsaturated fats are often derived from nuts or seeds and have more double bonds. Often people refer to saturated fats as bad, and monounsaturated and polyunsaturated fats as good. However, bear in mind that you do need some saturated fats in your diet. We just have to learn which ones are healthy.

The reason so many people need unsaturated fats is because the ratio between saturated and unsaturated is moderately out of balance in many modern-day diets, as was stated before. In the past, the foods that people consumed—even the animals used for food—were comprised of a good balance of saturated and unsaturated fats. Today, because of factory farming and convenience foods, most people have a higher intake of saturated fats, altered fats, and little or no intake of unsaturated fats. Because many Americans consume twenty times as much saturated fat as they do unsaturated, the average person in America, and in other countries, has a real need for the supplementation of the unsaturated fats, like omega-3 oils.

If saturated fats and unsaturated fats are out of balance, the body will not function normally. For example, saturated fats and omega-6 oils tend to increase our inflammatory response, which is a desirable thing when appropriate. If we consume primarily saturated fats, we may become hypersensitive, with our immune system stimulated unnecessarily. Unsaturated fats tend to slow down or mediate the immune response, which is also necessary. For health, we have to be able to initiate our defense system and use it, but we also have to be able to slow it down or stop it when the threat is dealt with. This is especially true with the immune system, since when people lose the ability to turn it off, they tend to develop autoimmune disease.

Essential fats are referred to as essential for a reason: they have to be consumed because the body cannot manufacture its own original source. Fatty acids are the basic building blocks of the body, and the body requires about twenty fatty acids in order to live and operate correctly. It can make limited amounts of many of these, except for linolenic and linoleic acid. These are the actual essential fatty acids that you must provide for your body. These fats tend to come from plant-based foods, especially nuts and seeds. Many seafoods are good sources of fats, since the algae consumed in the ocean is a good source for fats that many animals convert to a usable form for us. In some cases, there are people who have less ability to convert the essential fats, and seafood becomes a better source because the animals have already converted the fats to a usable form.

If the human cell is going to function correctly, the plasma cell membrane or outer barrier must be able to function properly too. If a human being is to be healthy, then a regular source of essential fats must be available. Many times fats are referred to by their "omega number." The omega number describes where the unbound carbon atom is located on the fat molecule. If that carbon atom is third from the end, the fatty acid is known as an omega-3 fatty acid. If it's sixth from the end, the fat is known as an omega-6 fatty acid. These fats tend to come from vegetables, nuts, and seeds. Omega-3 fatty acids have a valuable role in reducing the risk of inflammation, therefore avoiding an environment for heart disease and even cancer. The essential fatty acids are also important for building healthy brains and neural networks.

The fear of fat is therefore unjustified. Fat will not make you fat, and it is beneficial for your health as long as you consume good fats that are unaltered from natural sources. If you have not been consuming good fats, then start today. As soon as you introduce good fats, your body will be able to restore itself, and you will soon feel the difference. If you consume the right fats, you will actually lower your risk of breast cancer and colon cancer, improve learning and attention span, improve cognitive function, elevate moods and improve depression, lower the risk of cardiovascular disease, promote healthy skin, and even improve vision. You have the choice in the types of fats that you introduce into your own body. You can either choose healthy fats and create a vital functioning body, or you will live the consequences of the alternative.

The Good Fats

Naturally good fats are present in foods; they come from nature. For health, we have to strive for a balance of fat-type intake. Omega-3 essential fatty acids are polyunsaturated. These include alpha-linolenic acid (LNA), which comes primarily from plants; and eicosapentaenoic acid (EPA) and docosahexaenoic acid (DHA), which are obtained from animals like fish (and DHA from algae). When other animals consume plants, they convert LNA to DHA and EPA. If a person is a poor converter lacking important enzymes, this direct source provides an advantage.

Omega-6 essential fatty acids are polyunsaturated. Examples are Linoleic acid (LA), gamma linolenic acid (GLA), and arachidonic acid (AA). These are found in vegetable oils, nuts, and seeds. Omega-9 fatty acids are monounsaturated and include oleic acid, mead acid, and erucic acid. Saturated fats are also necessary and helpful, such as medium-chain triglycerides from virgin coconut oil. Most of us tend to get more saturated fat, and omega-6 predominant fats in our diet than we need, though.

Perhaps most important to brain function are linoleic (an omega-6 fatty acid) and alpha-linolenic acid (an omega-3). These become prime structural components of brain cell membranes and are also an important part of the enzymes within cell membranes that allow the membranes to transport valuable nutrients in and out of the cells. Also, one of the messengers sent by brain cells is a group of chemicals called prostaglandins. These are omega-6 fatty acids found in many oils, such as safflower, sunflower, corn, and sesame oils. Prostaglandins are also made with omega-3 fatty acids, which are found in flax, pumpkin seeds, walnuts, and cold water fish such as salmon and tuna.

Essential fatty acids are the fats least likely to make you fat. Essential fatty acids actually stimulate metabolism by speeding up the rate at which the body burns fat and glucose. In fact, many bodybuilders and fitness models will consume high-fat diets using medium-chain triglycerides in order to become very lean. In other words, you eat fat to lose fat.

Omega-3 fatty acids found in flax and fish oils also have the ability to act as a blood thinner. Remember that oils higher in monounsaturated and polyunsaturated fats will spoil more quickly. It is a good idea to consume antioxidants such as vitamin E, vitamin C, beta carotene, coenzyme Q10, which will prevent oils from going rancid. Cooking foods such as onions and garlic that are rich in antioxidants may lessen the damaging effect of heated oils.

A good fat, in my opinion, would have about 80 percent unsaturated fats and less than 20 percent saturated. As I mentioned before, many people are missing this component in their diet. It is interesting to note that human milk has the richest overall source of healthy fats. This makes good sense, since human milk is designed to help the baby develop a good nervous system, among other things. If you think about it, human milk is designed to grow an animal averaging about two hundred pounds of body weight with a very capable and large brain. Cow's milk, on the other hand, is designed to nurture an animal weighing an average of two thousand pounds, with limited brain capacity and size.

Algae oil is one of the richest sources of omega-3 fats, especially DHA.

Canola oil ranks second only to flax oil as an oil rich in essential fatty acids—again, especially DHA.

Soy products such as soy milk, tofu, tempeh, and edamame can be rich in essential omega-3 fats and omega-6 fatty acids similar to fish oils. The lecithin present in soy also helps reduce cholesterol and protects neural networks. However, be careful not to overdo soy, because of certain chemicals in soy like isoflavones that have the ability to interfere with normal hormones. There is also concern that genetically modified proteins in soy also pose a risk, and most of the soy we use is modified. The hormonal effect of soy isoflavones (hormone-like chemicals) can be a good tool, if a hormone like estrogen is dominant in the body. In this case, the soy isoflavones interfere with the excess estrogen and produce a calming response. On the other hand, you can create a weak hormone-like response or effect just like the presence of real hormones, if hormones are too low.

Note: plants contain chemicals that can mimic hormones, not real hormones. Sometimes plant fats are used to make hormones synthetically.

EPA and DHA from essential fats can be found in some plants, especially algae. For most healthy people, it is not hard to convert DHA to EPA. These are both important and essential fats. You can see also how animals who consume algae will also have a good balance of fats. When we eat other animals, we get the benefit of their protein, fats, and nutrient intakes. If the objective is to reduce inflammation and enhance nerve function, then we tend to use higher ratios of EPA. If our objective is to construct better tissues and networks, then we use a higher ratio of DHA.

DHA is the primary structural component of brain tissue. Research is increasingly recognizing the possibility that DHA has a crucial influence on neurotransmitters in the brain. Asian cultures have long appreciated the brain building effect of DHA. In Japan, DHA is considered such an important "health food" that it is used as a nutritional supplement to enrich some foods and students frequently take DHA pills before examinations.

Infants who have low amounts of DHA in their diet have reduced brain development and diminished visual acuity. The increased intelligence and academic performance of breast-fed children compared with formula-fed infants has been attributed in part to the increased DHA content of human milk. Cultures whose diet is high in omega-3 fatty acids (such as the Eskimos who eat a lot of fish) have a lower incidence of degenerative diseases of the central nervous system, such as multiple sclerosis. Experimental animals whose diets are low in DHA have been found to have smaller brains and delayed central nervous system development. Some children with poor school performance due to ADD have been shown to have insufficient essential fatty acids in the diet.

DHA is needed for healthy eyes. The more nutritious the fat, the better the eyes will function. Since most people are visual learners, better eyes produce better brains. Fats can also influence brain development and performance, especially at either end of life (e.g., growing infants and the elderly).

The most rapid brain growth is during the first year of life, with the infant's brain tripling in size. During this stage of rapid central nervous system growth, the brain uses 60 percent of the total energy consumed by the infant. Fats are a major component of the brain cell plasma membrane and of the myelin sheath built around each nerve. In fact, during the first year, around 50 percent of infants' daily calories come from fat.

Fat from fowl. Most fowl fat lies just under the surface of the skin. Once you remove the skin, the underlying meat is fairly lean, containing as low as 7 percent fat. Fowl that is truly free range will be rich in omega fatty acids. Eggs and meat from free-range chickens will contain more omega-3 fatty acids and a lower ratio of omega-6 to omega-3 fatty acids than factory- or cage-raised chickens.

The yolk of Greek eggs (which come from hens fed fish meal) contains six times the amount of omega-3 fat found in the usual US supermarket eggs. Similarly, ocean-caught wild fish contain more DHA than farm-raised fish do. This is because the fish eat algae, which is the primary producer of DHA on the entire planet.

Fish that swim and birds that run have healthier fat profiles than those in a cage or a pond. Muscle that exercises is leaner than muscle that just sits or floats. Also, plants that grow in the field or food that grows in the sea is nutritionally better than any factory-made foods. Farm-raised meat may contain as much as 40 percent more fat than free-roaming or free-swimming varieties.

The amount of DHA in a mother's breast milk is dependent on the amount of DHA in her diet. A recent study from Australia showed that infants nursing from others who had higher levels of DHA in their diets also had better mental development at one year of age. If the mother does not consume another DHA, the baby will actually steal from her brain to build its own.

Flaxseed happens to be one of the richest sources of essential fatty acids and does contain some DHA. The best way to consume flax oil is to use freshly ground flaxseeds, thereby having the freshest oil possible. Be wary of rancid oils; keep them at a cooler temperature and away from light. Fats are healthy for us in their natural state; however, once exposed even to the air or light, they can actually become unhealthy. A cheap coffee grinder will do a good job of grinding flaxseeds, and then you can sprinkle them on your food. You can buy flax oil or flax meal, but again, ensure that it is fresh and not spoiled. One caveat for flax oil: there are some studies linking high flax intake to prostate problems in males. It's not that males cannot consume flax oil, but high consumption may require some caution. Of course, flax for women is an excellent source of fats, and we do not know of a risk.

Fish and other seafood, especially cold-water types like salmon and tuna, are also excellent sources of unsaturated fats. It is theorized that because they live in cold water, they need a higher concentration of fats that remain liquid at colder temperature. Krill oil is highly regarded as a source of unsaturated fats. Fat from fish is nutritionally preferable because it is much higher in unsaturated fatty acids, whereas most animal fats are around 50 percent saturated and 50 percent unsaturated. Again, the animal's diet determines that ratio makeup.

Hummus, a popular food made from chickpeas and often with added tahini (crushed sesame seeds), has approximately 85 percent unsaturated fats, plus it is a fair source of protein, folate, and some vitamins and minerals. Even wheat germ can provide some good unsaturated fats.

Olive oil is a very valuable source of monounsaturated fats. It is an important component of the Mediterranean diet. Studies have demonstrated the Mediterranean diet to be one of the healthiest diets consumed. Nuts, like almonds and walnuts, can contain 90 percent unsaturated fats and some protein. Under-the-ground nuts like peanuts and cashews have lower unsaturated fat levels, but as I mentioned before, you do need some saturated fats. So peanuts can be a source of both saturated and unsaturated fats.

Some **plants** are rich sources of fat. Most plants do not contain a lot of fat, but what little they contain is high in essential fatty acids. Plants use omega-3 fatty acids to store the energy of sunlight. The darker and greener the leaves, the more essential fatty acids these leaves will usually contain.

Seeds, like sunflower, pumpkin, or borage seeds (and others), are a good source of omega-6 fatty acids. In fact, if you mix flax and borage oil, you receive a good mix of both omega-3 and omega-6 fats.

The Bad Fats

Bad fats contain a balance of saturated and unsaturated fatty acids. If eaten in moderation, they will contribute to your health and well-being. You may need to look for low-fat varieties, but these fat sources can be a rich source of other nutrients as well. I label them bad only because they contain a mix of saturated and unsaturated fats that is closer to 50-50.

Dairy products are mostly saturated fats, but this depends quite a bit on the diet of the animal. If the cow was grass fed and and lives a life more in line with natural animals, then the milk has a better concentration of unsaturated fats. However, most dairy consumed especially in this country comes from feedlot or dairy operations where the animal never consumes fresh grass. These are actually different animals in both their protein structure and the fat types available.

The most common milk consumed, if it is 1% or 2%, will have about half the fat content of whole milk. It is best if you know something about where your milk comes from. Dairy from healthy animals will have a healthier fat and protein profile.

Eggs—again, depending on how the animal is raised—will tend to have more or less unsaturated fat content. The yolk does tend to contain cholesterol, arachidonic acid, and other saturated fats. Overall, the egg is about 50-50 in its fat content, if you consume standard eggs.

Beef and other red meat is also about 50-50 in its ratio, if it is raised in feedlots on grains. Turkey also shares this ratio, as does veal and other red meat that is commonly consumed. However, let's say again that game meats and grass-fed beef have more health benefit without the risks.

Cocoa butter—even though the saturated fat has found to be very healthy if it is unprocessed. It contains medium-chain triglycerides, which are well utilized by the body and have health benefits.

The Ugly Fats

The ugly fats are those fats that really have no health value at all. You can eliminate all the fats in this category, and you would be healthier for it.

Any nutrient that might be contained in these fats is better obtained from other fat sources with better nutritional makeup. These are fats that have been altered by heat or exposure to air or light.

Fats in this category include **tallow** (chicken or beef) and 90 percent saturated fats like **lard**, which is high in saturated fatty acids. **Palm kernel oil**, which is mostly saturated fats, contains palmitoleic acid, a fat that, if eaten in excess, can interfere with essential fatty acid metabolism. **Margarines** are high in hydrogenated fats, especially those with a lot of palm kernel and other hydrogenated oils. **Shortening** can have large amounts of hydrogenated oils, palm kernel oils, coconut oils, or tallow. **Cottonseed oil** is more unsaturated than saturated, but it is usually found hydrogenated and may contain residues of pesticides.

Understand that there is a daily or circadian rhythm to life. This diurnal cycle is run basically by certain hormones. This daily cycle is often disrupted by altered fats. These altered fats (i.e., trans fats) are contained in most packaged foods. Butter, which tends to get a bad rap because of the saturated fat and cholesterol, has been replaced somewhat by margarine, which is also bad news for your health. When manufacturers chemically change food, many unanticipated problems occur, resulting in a dysfunctional body and poor health.

Remember, hydrogenated fats act differently biochemically in the body and interfere with structure and function. (Hydrogenation is one process used to create trans fats, but there are other processing methods.) Trans fats have been shown to raise LDL cholesterol and reduce the good, or HDL, cholesterol. Trans fats decrease the body's ability to reduce natural anti-inflammatory prostaglandins. The essential fatty acids are important for growth and function of vital organs, such as the brain, but altered fats are not essential. This has become a real concern, especially in children and frequent fast-food consumers whose daily diet is high in processed, deep-fried foods and snacks.

Trans fats interfere with the body's communication. They damage cell membranes, altering function. This means nutrients cannot get in, and waste products cannot get out. Plus, the receptors and antibodies on the surface of the membrane cannot be presented to do their job. This sets up the body for chronic degenerative diseases and dysfunction.

Remember that 60 percent of the brain and nerves are fat. The better the quality of fat in the diet, the better the brain and neural networks will function.

Chapter 5

Supplements

What Pill Do I Take for This?

Obviously, there is an overabundance of evidence indicating that medications of all kinds have helped suffering, given people a chance to reclaim their lives from disease, and of course have even saved lives. I fully acknowledge that drugs or medications play an important and necessary part in human culture and are positive tools to treat disease. Modern medications, when properly prescribed and used as directed, continue to be a positive development of our current society.

However, we must remember that drugs are produced for profit, and there are many conflicts of interest in their research and development. There is a quagmire of government regulation and government collusion with pharmaceutical manufacturers. Drugs also have their limitations, their unwanted side effects, and even life-threatening dangers. We must keep in mind that drugs are not necessarily designed or evaluated for long-term use. Medication produces as many negative, unwanted effects that produce disease because of its use alone, even to the extent of taking lives.

Again, I am not an anti-drug advocate. I believe that drugs, used appropriately, are an excellent tool and should be utilized whenever necessary. I also have witnessed that drugs can be limiting to health in their effects and tend to facilitate a sort of complacency. The majority of people utilizing medication tend not to focus on their own health, because they feel better with the drug, or even because of their belief that the drug has everything under control. Please don't be the person who assumes that they are healthy and can stop focusing on a solution to disease because a medication made the laboratory numbers look better. For example, someone may be placed on an acid-inhibiting drug because of indigestion or reflux. That same patient begins to assume that this means they now have license to eat any food that they want to. Generally, if you consume something that gives you indigestion, that substance should be avoided or taken differently. Don't use proton-pump inhibitors (acid-reflux drugs) to allow you to consume pizza and avoid symptoms.

What about the person without good control of blood sugar who takes a prescribed medication to control their blood glucose levels for them? This patient often assumes that the medication will control their blood sugar, so they don't have to watch what they eat and exercise. So this patient remains diabetic and under the management of the medical team, since they are doing nothing to correct their diabetes. If there are no lifestyle strategies, medications will never progress you toward health. I am not just singling out pharmaceutical medication here. I see just as many people with shopping bags full of nutritional supplements, herbs, and the latest do-it-quick pill. Medications and food supplements need to be used for a specific purpose to adjust or correct disease patterns. Perhaps an occasional multivitamin and multimineral might be used to make up for deficiencies common in our foods. We might make a case for the use of good fats such as fish and fish oils, since many people come up deficient. Probiotics are very important to our body function, and if we don't consume enough cultured foods, supplementation can help us to maintain a beneficial gut community.

In most cases, medications and nutraceuticals (concentrates and isolates of natural nutrients prescribed to help correct the disease process) are the short-term solution, used to keep things under control until you are ready and can resume better physiological functioning. There are a few examples where the drug or nutraceutical may be required for a longer period of time, and perhaps for an entire lifetime. However, most people using medications can make a choice to restore function by implementing a strategy of lifestyle changes. Remember that the great majority of drugs or medications have not even been studied for long-term use. These new-to-nature chemicals are designed to alter function, many times through interference or even stopping a process completely. This is done so that signs and symptoms can be decreased or controlled to ease suffering and allow the body some time to regenerate. It is up to you and your doctor to explore the mechanism that the medication is being used on, and then design a strategy to recover that mechanism, eventually solving the need for the drug.

When there is a good reason for using a medication or a nutritional supplement, by all means, gain the advantage. If a medication can keep you safe, then use it until, as soon as practical, you restore metabolic function and lower inflammatory processes. If you discover nutrient deficiency, or if you need to induce the body to do something it is not doing, choose and use the best nutraceutical cocktail that you can design. Many nutrients and natural chemicals can even improve physical capabilities and make a difference in athletic performance. Other natural chemicals are being discovered that can even increase longevity. I will even go so far as stating that I would much rather that you have expensive urine than experience the effects of a nutritional deficiency, as long as the substance in excess in your urine poses no danger to you. Natural chemicals and nutrients have the advantage of producing few if any side effects or damage.

However, even treatment with most nutraceuticals should have a strategy, and a defined time of use or an endpoint. What is the purpose for the vitamin, mineral, herb, concentrate, or precursor that you are taking? Are you dependent on it consistently, or do you just use it for a specific purpose? Concentrated nutrients and food supplements have the advantage of being able to restore function and correct mechanisms. Their effect seems to be more of moving the body toward better function by correcting mechanisms and systems instead of heavily shutting them down. Nutrients tend to affect several pathways at once, gently influencing systems, instead of focusing on one chemical pathway and interfering at one specific point, like medication does. Pharmaceutical drugs and even a "natural" pill need proper intent and monitoring of results. In other words, dependence is not a good outcome. Focus on lifestyle patterns first, and then supplements or perhaps medication as supplemental to a good diet. Health is self-sufficiency.

We are the most medicated society in history. Prescription drugs are the order of the day. People have their daily pill-supply system, and one must ask, what did humans do before they had all these pills? It is as if we had to wait to this point in our evolution so that someone could develop the new-to-nature molecule that would get the human body to actually work properly. The human body, if given sufficient care, can and will operate well on its own. If you find yourself organizing and scheduling your pill taking, think of how you could better use this time and money with a body that actually functions on its own.

I want you to consider especially how we are overmedicating the children. I have run across parents who use medications to put their young children to sleep, and then other medications to keep them alert and wake them up. We have young people experiencing diseases that in the past only occurred in the geriatric population. Drug makers are looking for even more applications for the use of their products in young children.

In truth, we have not yet adapted well to all this unnatural chemistry constantly introduced inside the human body. The body does a very good job on its own, if only given a chance without interference. All your body asks is that you avoid exposure to dangerous xenobiotics, allow the excretion of toxins if they gain entrance, and make sure you also get rid of your own physiological waste products. Your body requires that you take in an abundance of nutrients without an excess of calories, and maintain some level of physical activity. If a disease process becomes apparent, then the use of medication should be looked at solely as a tool. The medication allows the body systems to be under outside control while we restore function. When the human body functions properly, there is no disease, and more importantly, no longer a requirement for medication.

Whether we consider pharmaceutical drugs, herbs, homeopathic remedies, or even nutritional supplements, the key to health is not in a pill, potion, or cream. Health is created and maintained when you eat real food with a higher nutrient content and a lower calorie count. Give your body the nutrients that it needs and sufficient physical activity, and you will have long-term health and quality of life. If you ignore the factors that create a functional physiology, then you will need the interventions. Let's be clear about this: the medication strategy creates a dependency. It is just like putting on the little emergency spare tire in your car trunk. Then, instead of going to a tire supply store and replacing that tire with a good tire again, you decide to run around on the little spare, since it seems to work for the time being. Since you know that the car is designed to work with a much larger and better constructed tire, the best solution is to go get a new, proper tire. Would you intentionally attempt to walk and run by using a crutch even after your leg is healed? The crutch was a temporary solution until you could use your leg again, just like the medication.

But if you listen to the media, there seems to be that everlasting promise that there's now a pill that will make you look better, feel better, lose weight, be stronger, and be smarter. The only strategy that really delivers consistently is your lifestyle. Let us remember that drugs exist to make money for the shareholders of pharmaceutical companies. Profits drive many more important decisions than research or medical treatment outcomes. What is in your best interest may not always be in line with what is in the best interest of the company providing you medication. Keeping this in mind, I suggest that we utilize the minimum amounts of medication necessary for what we are trying to accomplish. Ask questions and understand what the medication you are taking is for. Ask what you should expect to get from this drug, and also what side effects there may be. I encourage you to ask this of your prescribing physician, but also to have a detailed discussion with the pharmacist.

If you are currently not dependent on any medication, then consider what your strategy will be to absolutely minimize the need for such treatment. If you currently use or are prescribed a pharmaceutical drug, then what is your strategy for eventual freedom and self-sufficiency? It is up to you to learn what the drug does for you and exactly why you are taking it. Is the drug alleviating certain symptoms? Is the drug being used because of some finding on lab work? What is the reason for each particular prescription, whether by a practitioner or by your own choice to use? What is the mechanism that this drug is affecting? How can you correct, stop, or enhance that same mechanism without the drug? As you look into the drug and its effects, you will likely find that lifestyle factors can and do make huge differences as well. For example, most mechanisms that are affected by drugs are also very affected by exercise. In many cases, the right type of activity will make a significant difference and even resolve many health problems. Your symptoms, if you are overweight, will commonly be alleviated by changes in body composition. Fat deposition in fat cells creates an entire endocrine organ capable of producing hormones, immune system modulators, and even neurotransmitters.

Supplements can be helpful as well, but look for supplements that are making a positive difference in function. When you are under stress, you may need more of an essential nutrient because the stress response is using more of the B vitamin family, as an example. This is referred to as "conditionally essential" requirements, which may happen with nutrients that your body can produce but under certain conditions will require more. Dr. Jeffrey Bland has proposed that even oxygen is conditionally essential under certain conditions. Sometimes if I can just get a patient to learn to breathe, problems disappear. Sleep apnea, lack of physical activity, low blood pressure, and many other situations render people oxygen deprived. I am proposing that you look to the essential items first, such as oxygen. The need for the rest may take care of itself.

Weight Loss, Supplements, and Dependency

Some supplements used are thermogenic, creating heat and raising the body's metabolism as their effect. This can be helpful for weight loss as long as the body is stimulated properly and burns mostly fat. Thermogenesis, the production of heat, results in increased burning of calories. Some supplements are based on the thermogenic effects of caffeine. Many supplements have used ephedrine, and there are numerous other herbs that produce a thermogenic or calorie-burning effect. One of the best thermogenics that we use in our clinic comes from an extract of chili peppers. This can be used for a more energetic feeling as well; however, I caution you not to create an overdependence on these stimulants.

Other supplements can block the absorption of carbohydrates in the stomach and intestine, such as wheat amylase starch or certain fibers like the konjac root. There are also supplements and drugs that block the absorption of fat, but I do not recommend these. Fat blockers can be somewhat annoying and even dangerous, since they will block the absorption of certain important nutrients and generally cause a lot of digestive upset and even explosive diarrhea. There are supplements, herbs, and drugs that can suppress your appetite, and of course some are safer than others. There are substances and medications that can help to regulate thyroid function. This can be helpful, because as people go through starvation diets, there is an entire resetting of thyroid function. When this happens, metabolism slows down and fat is more readily accumulated.

Any stress response will block the metabolism of fat. Your body's major stress response comes from the immune system. Many people are sensitive to certain foods and chemicals that stimulate an immune response, thereby impairing fat burning. It is becoming more prevalent for people to experience a process called autoimmunity, where the immune system begins to attack tissues in the body. If this is directed at the thyroid gland, it will create a dysfunction of the thyroid, eventually leading to the accumulation of weight. Commonly, gluten sensitivity is implicated in this process. This is referred to as Hashimoto's thyroiditis, eventually creating hypothyroidism.

I'm sure that you've also heard about cortisol and its effect on weight control. When cortisol levels are high for extended periods of time, your body will preferentially use other fuel sources aside from fat. Cortisol will facilitate the breakdown of muscle while impairing the use of your fat stores, so that you utilize protein from the muscles for your energy. So controlling cortisol can be a real help for weight loss as well keeping you healthy. But understand that cortisol is an important corticosteroid hormone, and you need the right amount at the right times for your daily functioning. Cortisol and melatonin run your day and night cycle. Cortisol awakens you in the morning; melatonin puts you to sleep at night. If cortisol levels run too high or too low, your sleep is affected, and you will struggle with weight control.

Most of the drugs used for weight loss do not have a good track record for safety. Although this is the most popular way to lose weight, prescription medication for weight loss holds hidden dangers. There is a long list of side effects and risks when utilizing many of the drugs prescribed for weight loss. Heart disease, liver and kidney damage, and even cancer are described as possible risks. In fact, the risks are too great in my opinion for the small amount of weight loss that will likely be accomplished. It is interesting that many of the drugs used for weight loss failed to be safe enough for their original application, but since they altered metabolism or reduced appetite, they were approved for weight loss.

Bariatric surgery certainly isn't a supplement, but it's become a popular approach to weight loss. Although some people claim to have done well with bariatric surgery, there are also serious risks to consider. Of course there is the risk of complications from any surgery, and this must be taken into account. With bariatric surgery, you are making physical alterations to the structure of your digestive system. Studies have demonstrated that this alteration also increases your risk of autoimmune disease, alcoholism, and neurological and brain disorders. This makes sense if you understand that a large part of the immune system is incorporated into your gastrointestinal tract. When you start altering your digestive system, you also make large alterations to your immune system and its response. You also change how well nutrients are absorbed. Bariatric surgery has recently been touted as a treatment for diabetes. In my opinion, this is a very extreme measure when simple dietary changes and exercise are even more effective, without the danger.

One study indicated that diabetes was better resolved with surgery, but diet changes quickly caught up. The truth is that is most people who undergo bariatric surgery find ways to get around the physical alterations. All the surgery does is create a situation where you physically can't eat as much. The procedure does nothing to help you make better choices or to live a healthier life. The surgery is really nothing more than forcing starvation. Again, in my years of experience, the most effective thing that I have seen people do is simply to make better choices in food. If you choose to eat the right kind of foods, then you don't have need of calorie counting or extreme surgical procedures.

You can find programs where meals are prepared for you, and therefore control what you eat, but someday you have to learn to be self-sufficient again. You are also trusting that the manufacturer or preparer of the meals is giving you something that is actually healthy. If you have the luxury of a personal chef, or if you wish to purchase pre-prepared meals, just ensure that you are getting the same foods that I hope you would prepare for yourself. There are also bars, drinks, and many herbal concoctions that are used to aid people in losing weight. Some are generally regarded as safe; others can be hazardous to you. Just like choosing fresh, whole, organic, and nutritious foods when you shop, apply the same criteria to whatever prepackaged products you will consume. Try to avoid "snack bars," and instead choose food bars that contain wholesome nutrients and sufficient protein. Ideally, 14 to 30 grams of protein, along with other actual food ingredients, make the best choice. Pay attention to the amount of added sugar, binders, fillers, and preservatives. The same goes for drink mixes: make good judgments and ensure that you are consuming something that will benefit you.

The most effective thing that you will ever do to maintain your weight is to maintain your health. Strive to be a vital, happy person by primarily consuming these real foods. I do not see people struggle to maintain their weight or health when they are consuming primarily vegetables, a small amount of fruit, and good sources of protein. I have seen time and time again that the person who consumes real food does not even have to pay close attention to calorie intake or portion control. There are a few supplement ingredients that I would consider safe to use (see list below). You can look for these in the ingredient listing; however, pay attention to everything else which is included in the supplement that you have chosen. Purchase from a company that you can trust and do your homework. You might go so far as to contact the company and ask for a product assay to have more confidence that the active ingredients are present in amounts that would be beneficial.

Recommended Supplements

If you are curious about what supplements you should take, I suggest you keep it to a minimum. First, we can make a case for the utilization of a good *multivitamin and multimineral* product because of our food's nutrient depletion and the fact that most of us are not consuming the greatest diet. When we do laboratory testing, we tend to find various deficiencies. I would also suggest supplementing *good fats,* since the majority of people tend to require more unsaturated fats than they get in their diet. When we test people for essential fats, we again often find deficiencies. The third supplement I would recommend would be *probiotics.* Yes, you can consume some foods that contain cultures; however, most of us have a need for ongoing supplementation. The beneficial and commensal organisms that we carry with us can be reduced or destroyed with such things as antibiotics. Probiotics protect us: they help us digest and help to regulate our immune response.

Any other supplement that I might recommend on top of a good diet would be for a specific purpose, to address signs of dysfunction or symptoms and provide something that we found lacking in reviewing laboratory testing. If you are working on a healthy weight-loss strategy, here are some clinically researched ingredients. The following substances have actually been tested in clinical trials and were found to be safe and at least somewhat effective.

Beta–methoxy–phenylethylamine is actually considered a neurotransmitter. It is often tested as a gauge for brain function. You do not want the level of this substance too high in the body, since we know it is related to attention-deficit disorder and hyperactivity. It is also effective at enhancing metabolic rate and fat burning.

Pyruvate is an intermediate product of the Krebs cycle, and if you feed more into the system, the cycle will feed forward. What this means is that your energy production and fat burning can be enhanced. Since it is a normal byproduct of metabolism, it is actually very safe to use, and you will find it in many products, especially among the bodybuilding crowd.

Conjugated linoleic acid (CLA) is actually a natural trans fat that was first discovered along with colostrum in cow's milk. Presently it is manufactured using fats such as safflower oil. It is actually one of the few healthy trans fats and has been well studied in both immunotherapy and sports medicine. This substance seems to greatly enhance fat burning if the person is doing intense exercise. Interestingly, it is not found to be very effective for people who are not physically active.

L-carnitine is an amino-acid derivative used by the body to transport fat into the cells and therefore enhance fat metabolism. The dosage needs to be high enough for the effect (usually about 3 grams), but it is a well-studied and well-known supplement for sports performance and even weight loss.

Dehydroepiandrosterone (DHEA) is the major steroid hormone produced by the adrenal glands. It is also produced by the gonads and the brain. DHEA is the most abundant circulating steroid hormone. It can act by itself both directly and through its metabolites, which include androstenediol and androstenedione. It can then be further converted to testosterone and estrogens. Since DHEA is a precursor of many important hormones, it is also neuroprotective. DHEA has been found to have many more beneficial effects.

In some cases, some supplementation can be very helpful to supply more DHEA to the body, and in other cases adding DHEA can correct certain pathways that may be imbalanced. For example, a situation called pregnenalone steal can redirect the pathway involving DHEA, and supplementation can restore balance. Supplementation may also be effective in neural degenerative diseases.

DHEA in the 7-Keto form has also been found to enhance fat loss. In this format it will not affect hormones, but it does affect the Krebs cycle and fat burning.

The **ECA stack** is a very popular combination in the bodybuilding culture. This is a combination of ephedrine, caffeine, and aspirin. These three substances seem to have a synergistic effect on fat-burning energy. This popular stack is used by many bodybuilders to get very lean before competition and also to have more intense workouts.

Nitric oxide is currently a very popular molecule. It is being studied because of its effect on circulation and treatment for heart disease and hypertension. Enhancing the production of nitric oxide can be very helpful in building muscle, increasing fitness, and even burning fat. There are certain amino acids and amino acid derivatives that increase the production of nitric oxide. This has a very beneficial effect on circulation, as it helps blood vessels to open. Currently there is a lot of study on nitric oxide and cardiovascular function. It is currently being utilized as a treatment for heart disease. Because of the effect of nitric oxide, you will also enhance overall blood circulation, build muscle faster and more effectively, and even enhance sexual function in males and females.

Alpha lipoic acid (ALA) is a fascinating molecule. You can produce it in your body; however, taking a certain amount as a supplement can really increase the benefits. ALA is a fantastic antioxidant and is able to recharge itself. It has great benefits that contribute to a successful healthy aging strategy, as well as positive effects on blood sugar and regeneration of cells. A lot has been done using ALA to protect and regenerate the liver. It does a great job in helping people to regulate their metabolism, and it can enhance energy production even to the point of stimulating the production of mitochondria, which are your fuel cells. I mention it here because it can also help in weight control.

Fucoxanthin is an antioxidant found naturally in edible brown seaweed such as wakame, the seaweed used in miso soup. Studies in animals suggest that this substance will help the body target abdominal fat, the visceral fat that is more dangerous to accumulate. It is one of the things being credited for the longevity, health, and weight control of the Okinawan people. Their consumption of seaweed apparently has many benefits.

Hoodia is an herb that is a natural appetite suppressant, but you have to make sure that the supplement form that you take has the active ingredients. If the hoodia is not grown in harsh desert conditions, where it was originally found, it doesn't produce the active ingredients that will suppress the appetite effectively. This is something to consider with all supplements, since they are not regulated as closely as pharmaceuticals. The safety of nutritional supplements and herbs is very high, but many companies unintentionally may use sources of lesser quality. Some supplements have even been tested and found not to contain things printed on the label.

Guarana is a plant native to the Amazon forest. It has black seeds that are rich in caffeine, and as stated before, caffeine does have benefits for weight loss by creating thermogenesis.

Chromium is a mineral needed for normal carbohydrate, fat, and protein metabolism. It is an important component of the hormone insulin and has been found in clinical studies to promote weight loss and control blood sugar and diabetes. Even though it is considered a micronutrient and we only need a very small amount, it has been found that many people are deficient.

Apple cider vinegar has a reputation for many health benefits and also acts as an appetite suppressant. It enhances digestion and can be used as a natural cleaner, also improving pH in the body. It is considered an effective supplement for weight loss.

Chitosan is a supplement derived from crustacean shells, such as crab shells. It has a demonstrated effect on fat absorption. Digestive problems have been reported in many people, and this is true of most fat blockers. Better to choose good fats and taken important nutrients with them.

Ma huang (ephedra sinica) is a plant native to Asia that contains natural ephedrine. The substance was banned for a period of time because of its relationship to heart attacks. However, if the correct dosage is used, this is a very safe substance. It has recently been allowed back on the market, and its effects on increasing metabolic rate are helpful for weight loss.

Bitter orange (citrus aurantium) is an herb somewhat similar to ephedra. It contains compounds similar to ephedrine and is used for similar effects.

These are just a few substances used and studied for weight loss. There are also other acceptable supplements, but keep in mind that supplements cannot accomplish your health goals. They may be helpful to shed a few pounds, induce physiological effects, or even help the body move toward healthy function, but there is nothing more effective than consuming real food and getting sufficient physical activity. That is the theme of this book. In the eternal search for shortcuts to success in health, nothing can outperform the way that you choose to live your life.

Part Two

Get Physically Active

Chapter 6

The Case for Physical Activity

How would you like to experience a complete transformation of your body—a true metamorphosis into a body that looks better, feels better, and in reality works better? It is quite possible to create a new and different body for you to live in instead of just altering your appearance. Consider all the money and effort people put into "creating a look." Of course everyone wants to look good, and looking better requires some effort. If you have the desire to look better, the proven secret is to feel better. When you're healthy and when you feel good, you will look like a completely different person. The most effective thing you can do for a celebrity physical appearance is to create and maintain your health. The human body contains an invaluable characteristic: it can regenerate and actually reinvent itself. Biologically it is possible to make your body younger than your years. If you understand the concept of transformation, and you understand the human body, then you won't need nearly as much of the artificial appearance enhancers.

I encourage you to strive for real health instead of only the appearance of health.

The human body is designed and evolved to move. Exercise and physical activity keep your biological systems working and maintain, even strengthen, the tissues of your body. If you suffer an injury, you can rehabilitate that injury and most of the time end up better off than you were before. Your physical appearance and your mental function are both improved when you are physically active.

The human body never makes a mistake. Your body is a collection of biological systems that are only responding to how you go about living your life. When you are physically active, you facilitate the construction of a body that can better handle whatever physical activity you engage in. This is called physical adaptation, and it is an ongoing process throughout your lifetime. As long as you don't overwhelm, overstress, or over train the body, this adaptive change will be a positive thing.

When you use your body through being physically active, you create a body that is bigger, faster, stronger, and smarter. Your neural network, your brain, your nervous system, and every little nerve fiber in your body will be better if it is used. The current theory of how we learn is actually based on how much we use certain parts of our nervous system and our brain. Use nerves by being physically and mentally active, and this will increase the trophic flow of nutrition to that nerve. The nerve actually grows larger and carries the signals better. Continue to use that nerve, and a myelin sheath is built around the nerve. The sheath is an insulator, but it also facilitates better quality and faster nerve signals along the myelin itself. As we mentioned before, this is how we learn a skill: we facilitate a certain neural network and get better at performing a movement, or even at thinking or recalling memories.

If you are physically active, you will have stronger muscle, bone, ligaments, and enhanced circulation. There are two well-known laws of human physiology. *Wolff's law* has to do with the remodeling of bone and states that bone in animals will adapt to the loads placed upon it. High bone density does not necessarily mean strong bones. Taking extra calcium and other nutrients, or perhaps taking medication or hormones that maintain bone density, only ensures denser bone. Strong bone contains a collagen trabecular structure with the density of bone mineralization around it. Bone density without bone structure turns out to be weak and brittle. If you want strong bones, you must place appropriate stress on the bones, and they will model their structure according to that stress. Weight-bearing exercise is the most effective method of creating strong bones.

In physiology, *Davis's law* describes how soft tissue models according to imposed stresses and demand. Muscle, tendon, and ligament will remodel and adapt to any load placed upon them. It is interesting that in studies of Paleolithic and early man, scientists have found much stronger bone structure, indicating that early man was much more physically powerful than we are today. We are less active than our predecessors, and we have become at least physically inferior to our ancestors. Many people, even over the short span of a few generations, have actually become weaker beings. In current society, people experience more sarcopenia (loss of muscle mass) and weaker bones than even a few generations ago. However, body structure can differ significantly depending on how physically active each person is. We do have some people in our society living in very healthy and strong bodies that can physically and mentally function at a higher level. The differences are only partially genetic; in fact, most of the differences between people occur because of what we do day to day.

In our clinic, we utilize testing of physical fitness and physiological parameters. I find in each study that the people who are physically active in their daily lives are much more physically fit, as you might imagine. What stands out is that these active people actually have a completely different physiology that can be measured. For example, a person who has been physically active tends to have a physiology that more readily accesses and burns fat. A person more sedentary becomes more dependent on dietary carbohydrates and is more efficient at storing fat. Your lifestyle actually creates the fat burner or the sugar burner. This is not a genetic thing; it is simply related to the person's activities of daily living. The evidence for this is that everyone I have worked with has been able to change their lifestyle, thereby shifting this physiology.

If you're physically active, you tend to alleviate and even negate the physically damaging effects of stress. We understand that under stress, your body is getting ready for a physical fight or a physical flight. If you don't move, the same response will still occur and actually begin to damage your body. If you feel constantly under stress, this is a condition referred to as sympathetic dominance. In this case, not only is this damage from stress ongoing, but you never enter an effective repair and recovery phase. Your autonomic nervous system is designed to operate utilizing a sympathetic as well as a parasympathetic system. If you cannot effectively enter or utilize the parasympathetic system, then you will not be able to effectively sleep, digest, recover, or even be able to perform as well sexually. Physical activity activates the sympathetic system and then automatically transitions to the parasympathetic system. You very likely need exercise to facilitate this transition, and it is your only option for recovery.

If you want a makeover, you can utilize clothing that makes you look like you are in better shape then you really are. With new fabrics available, it has become very popular to wear "slimming undergarments"—a little more advanced and effective than the corset was. We use lotions, creams, lasers, Botox, and even surgery to look different on the outside. Think of all the personal care products used, even perhaps plastic surgery considered, to alter the outward appearance of someone's body. I encourage you to take better care of yourself. Instead of this artificial alteration of physical appearance, I suggest thinking in terms of a true change and transformation. Truly, you can create a new and better body to experience life in.

There is nothing wrong with the practice of cosmetology, and in fact, we even offer certain procedures at our wellness clinic. People don't have to stop using personal care products that are safe, or many of the procedures that people use at home for both hygiene and appearance. There is also a place for practitioners to help you improve your appearance and your health if you are disfigured or exhibit the results of poor health. This might entail cosmetic surgery, or the help of a dermatologist.

However, don't abandon effective strategies that you can set up for yourself. Physical fitness and physical beauty truly are generated from within. The most effective method for flawless skin and a body that looks, feels, and performs well is within everyone's grasp. It does take time, and it does take effort, but there is nothing like the real thing. If you practice good nutrition, proper and effective exercise, and live in the cleanest environment possible, the results will be dramatic. For many people, the word "exercise" intimidates or frustrates them. For others, even though they are aware of the benefits, they have told themselves that they don't have time. It can be effective to start with small amounts of activity throughout your day. You could walk further and walk more frequently. It will pay off greatly if you start scheduling time to incorporate physical activity. Make it a priority, because it is just that important. If you let your health go, then what else matters? If you have not been physically active, than assess yourself and get started at the level that you're at right now. If walking around the block is challenging, then start with a fraction of the block and continue to work on more distance. Be careful not to fall into the trap of believing that you are so fragile that you cannot exercise. Just do it; just get started.

Incorporate consistency into your exercise routine. Physical activity must occur on an ongoing basis. A few minutes here and there or an exhaustive workout once a week, although they may create some benefit, will not be near as effective. Women especially require consistent, daily physical activity to maintain weight and to realize the benefits of exercise. You really do not need a "rest day" as long as there is variety in your workout routine. I suggest that you plan exercise for most days of the week. A day or two of rest a week should be sufficient. When your exercise reaches an exhaustive intensity, then rest days will be planned. For most people not engaged in competition-level training, it is best to find a way to plan activity into your daily routine. Most workouts are effective for a time window of about 40 to 60 minutes. Some more intense workouts will have benefit even in 20-to-30-minute windows. The exception to this would be building endurance, which may require a longer workout.

Yes, you can do too much exercise. With overtraining your improvement is limited, and you will find it harder to recover. Human beings generally can work at their peak for about 60 minutes. This does not mean that you cannot exercise beyond an hour, but there may be diminishing returns. There are African hunters who have been known to run down their prey, running nonstop for up to 16 hours. The endurance athletes who do ultra-long events have trained to perform for these long periods of time. Human physiology tends to keep enough glycogen, or stored sugar, for about an hour's worth of intense activity. Beyond that time, the body must rely more on fat stores and the use of other body tissues like muscle, and even bone and organ.

Create a challenge. If your exercise is not challenging to you, then there's no stimulus for the body to adapt and improve. To really benefit from physical activity, you must push yourself outside of your comfort level, but not push yourself to the point of overtraining. Overtraining often results in injury and creates a situation where you are not ready for your next workout because your body needs more time to recover. You can push yourself without creating injury or experiencing fatigue. This concept requires that you determine what level is your baseline. If you would struggle to simply walk around the block, then you must determine what you are capable of and present yourself a challenge slightly beyond that. Perhaps you start with a walk to the end of the block, with the goal of progressing to going around the entire block. I also want you to ignore the saying "no pain, no gain." When you perform exercises such as weight training, the objective is not soreness. Although you may experience soreness, especially upon starting a new or different routine, what you are looking for is the adaptation.

If your exercise is not challenging, then you are not going to make gains. As you continue to do only what your body is already adapted to, then you will produce little or no results. Sure, you might burn a few calories, you might even break a sweat, but you are not going to create a new and better body. I have worked with innumerable people who were totally invested in their daily walk on the treadmill. They had been told to do low-intensity exercise and stay in the fat-burning zone. These people often were seeing weight gain, fatigue, and illness, because they were not training their body to burn fat better and actually ended up burning muscle for energy. I've also worked with many bodybuilders and endurance athletes who will perform an intense workout, improve their physical performance, and yet experience no muscle soreness or fatigue whatsoever.

If you only do one thing towards creating health in mind and body, I would suggest that you find a way to become more physically active. Exercise seems to be the first thing to drop when you're busy. Either people get busy, or they don't want to make the effort, or perhaps for some other reason people just decide to stop being physically active. Our daily lives don't require physical exertion the way they used to. Very few people have jobs or activities that incorporate any physical exertion at all. Even people who work in an industry that used to require physical labor now find themselves in most cases sitting in a truck or on a tractor or even at a desk. Perhaps modern living has become (at least physically) too easy and convenient. Yet exercise and producing energy are likely the most important things that your body can do.

You can't wait for the energy to show up before you start exercising. The production of energy is a response to the activities and needs of your body. The energy production of the human body is directly related to the intensity, duration, and type of physical activities performed. When you exercise, your body begins to adapt so that it can meet the energy demands. The converse is true as well: when your life is sedentary, energy does not increase; it actually decreases.

Energy production takes place in cells called mitochondria. These are your little fuel cells that provide energy for you. It was once thought, and is still theorized, that the mitochondria were separate and distinct organisms from us, and then infected our cells, or joined us. They were good at producing energy and became our primary energy source. When you are less active, there is less need for energy to be produced. The mitochondrion then begins to atrophy, shrinking in size, and eventually some will die.

This means you will actually lose mitochondria or, more often, at least impair their function. When you exercise, the result is the opposite, and your mitochondria will increase in size, number, and efficiency of energy production. This is "use it or lose it" in action: use your body, or atrophy and degeneration will occur.

Recently, more information has been discovered concerning the pathways that produce mitochondrial increases in size, efficiency, and number. One of these pathways is called the SIRT 1 pathway. This pathway is stimulated by certain nutrients in the body and by exercise. Resveratrol, alpha lipoic acid, nitric oxide, and other molecules are able to facilitate this pathway. Without the stimulation of physical activity, though, there is not as great of an impact. With physical activity, there is rapid growth of size and number of mitochondria. When this occurs, you are literally producing more energy more efficiently, and you will feel the difference.

The best motivation for exercise is when you experience the adaptive changes and all the benefits. When you exercise with enough intensity so that you feel challenged, you will stimulate the adaptation, or change. If you live a more sedentary lifestyle, the results are fatigue and the degenerative changes that many usually blame on aging. A sedentary lifestyle coupled with the lack of good nutrition (getting the necessary nutrients) creates the average American person. These people are tired, overweight, dependent upon numerous medications, and expending a lot of money and effort going to doctor's visits. Things don't just happen to you; they are created as a result of a sequence of events or a mechanism. The mechanism of energy production is very important, since as soon as energy is depleted, the human body cannot function. What is your strategy? How are you preparing to avoid the loss of healthy function and energy?

Chapter 7

Effective Exercise

There are numerous types of exercise, and even though people like to claim that one is better than the other, to some extent they all have benefits if done correctly. I suggest that you design a workout program that utilizes different types of exercise to take advantage of all the benefits. The only way to build a more functional body is to ensure that you have physical strength and stability, as well as aerobic capacity, balance, range of motion, endurance, and coordination. Training the body properly creates demand for a better body, and the good news is the body has the capacity to create, rebuild, regenerate, and restore itself if you request that. You can reinvent your own body.

Resistance Training

It is best to invest some time building strong tissue around joints. Ligaments and muscles function to provide movement and stability. If joints themselves are not strong and stable, you will have ongoing problems with your joints. The direct way to create new muscle, bones, tendons, ligaments, and nerves, and even enhance the function of internal organs, is to apply the proper physical stresses. With resistance training, you can strengthen and stabilize joints while you create a more powerful and attractive body. Power is the ability to do things, and you must create a structure that can translate that power into some form of action. Power is not necessarily based on size alone. Men and women can be very powerful and strong without gaining the size sought after in bodybuilding.

A big problem in our modern society is people that are in a state of sarcopenic obesity. They have unknowingly experienced a loss of muscle over time. These are people who look okay but are really overfat. These skinny-but-fat people, usually over time, have lost a great deal of muscle and gained some fat. Muscle and other tissue is not static but is ever-changing, either being broken down as a protein source or maintained and built as adaptation. To maintain muscle mass, you must stimulate the growth of new muscle constantly. Studies indicate that even at the level of your DNA, where protein synthesis originates, the body needs some kind of a signal. If the amount of resistance or stress placed upon a muscle is sufficient, or is somewhat challenging and beyond what the body is used to, then protein synthesis is begun and new muscle is built.

This does require a fair amount of stress. Simply lifting a very light weight for a high number of repetitions has been determined to be more of an aerobic workout and does not produce significant muscle gain. If you use a mid to low range of repetitions, while utilizing more weight, then your body will begin the synthesis of muscle at the level of your DNA.

Exercises are done in *sets*, which consist of a number of *repetitions* (reps), or times that the exercises are performed. I recommend working in a repetition range of 6 to 12 and doing 3 to 6 sets of each exercise. In the beginning, a good way to set how much weight to use is to determine the maximum weight that you can use and still be able to perform the number of repetitions planned. If you plan on a set of 10 repetitions, then choose a weight that you can perform those repetitions with good form only 10 or maybe 11 times. If you can continue beyond the planned number of repetitions, then you need more weight. On the other hand, if you choose a weight that is too heavy and you cannot do all of your planned repetitions, then you need a lighter weight.

There are many variations that can be performed as well. *Supersets* are done with one exercise following another, often opposing, muscle group. *Giant sets* are combinations of more than two exercises following on another. Sometimes an entire circuit is done with several exercises in a sequence. There are numerous designs of weight machines, and although they can be effective, they tend to isolate muscles and can train a less natural motion. I prefer to mix in some free weights for the intrinsic stabilization muscles to be recruited.

There are other ways to choose how much weight to use, based on one repetition maximum or fatigue (failure) or eccentric contraction movements, but this is used more for advanced weight training. If you work out a plan of mid-range repetitions, with the heaviest weight with which you can maintain form and technique, you will build muscle. There is also a system called high-intensity training where fewer repetitions are performed and the exercise is done very slowly. This can also be an effective method. The objective is not to "bulk up," build massive muscles, or even become a power lifter. The objective is to build and maintain a normal amount of muscle mass. The objective is also to have joints that are strong enough and stable enough for the activities of life that you want to do.

Weight training has always been considered to be anaerobic exercise only, although it also helps you aerobically while maintaining or increasing muscle. As mentioned earlier, each type of exercise that you do predominates in one major benefit, while also providing other adaptations or benefits to a lesser extent. For most of us, I do not recommend weight lifting every day. In fact, we can do quite well utilizing weights one, two, or three times a week depending on our objectives. I propose that you plan some form of exercise for most days of the week, if not every day. If you're not doing seriously intense training for some competition, you will not necessarily need rest days. It is also a fact that even the best of athletes have about an hour's worth of peak performance available to them at a time. This does not mean the well-trained athlete cannot perform for longer periods, but we also have to take into account human physiology and energy storage.

For maximum benefit in training, with the exception of training for endurance, workouts should not last much over an hour, especially if they are intense. Sometimes a workout is effectively done in half of that time. This is why the triathlete will split a routine into smaller workouts—maybe a morning session and then an evening session with different types of training. That way, with a few hours of recovery in between, they can accomplish training in the different modes of exercise. If your goal is to be healthy, then I am suggesting that you incorporate weight training for all of its benefits. But as we go on here, you will see that there are other forms of exercise that are just as important. The most effective exercise is the exercise in which you invest your full focus and intensity. Make every workout pay you a dividend so that you don't waste time.

Aerobic Exercise

In additional to resistance training, it is important to enhance your aerobic capacity, and this is something that can be measured in the clinic and by improvements in performance. In our clinic, we measure oxygen uptake ($V0_2$ max). By measuring the amount of oxygen you consume during exercise, we can correlate that to how much fuel you can burn and how powerful you are during physical activity.

Interval Training

The most effective way to train to increase aerobic capacity is called *interval training*. There are several variations of this type of training. Intervals can be done on equipment, such as the treadmill or stationary cycle, or it can be done outside running, cycling, or swimming. The mistake that I want you to avoid is simply getting on the treadmill at a slow speed without incline (low intensity) and listening to music or watching TV. If you want the exercise to pay off, focus on training intervals of high intensity alternating with much lower-intensity recovery phases (such as wind sprints).

If you are injured, are just beginning, have no exercise capacity, or just want a clear head, then walk. Honestly, if this is all you can really do right now, then that is appropriate for you. When you're ready to move ahead and actually increase fitness, then start interval training, even if this is simply walking slower and then walking faster. To do interval training, first warm up for five to ten minutes at a low intensity. After warming up, perform a very intense period followed by a recovery period, and repeat this routine. For example, you might start with two-minute intervals on a treadmill. For two minutes, manually set the treadmill to the highest speed and increase to the maximum incline that you keep up with, pacing yourself for two full minutes. After that, reduce the treadmill in speed and drop the incline to zero, and spend two minutes recovering at a very easy pace but not stopping completely.

There are various ways to perform interval training. What you are attempting to do is to challenge yourself for a short period of time based on your current capabilities. Then you want your body to be allowed to recover, and this is just as important. Anybody can utilize intervals, because they should always be based on a challenging but not overwhelming physical exertion, followed by a low-intensity recovery. One effective way to determine how many intervals to do is to watch the recovery of your heart after each interval.

If you have a heart rate monitor, you can watch, according to time, the rate at which your heart rate is decreasing while you are in the recovery time period. If you don't have a heart rate monitor, you can take your own pulse. Simply count your pulse for five seconds every other five-second period of time. You are waiting for a difference in recovery to occur. As long as your heart rate goes up and comes down at the same steady pace, you will continue to do further intense intervals. At some point you will notice that your heart rate is not coming down as quickly as before, and this is the point at which you will stop the intervals. I recommend after that you spend about twenty minutes cooling down, just spend twenty minutes at a nice easy pace, letting your body recover from the interval training. The intense intervals may only last ten to fifteen minutes, or sometimes thirty minutes or more.

Endurance Training

It is as important to repair the body by training to improve its endurance capabilities. There are many ways to do this; however, if you are going to train for endurance, you have to put your body in a situation where it doesn't have much choice but to burn fat better for a longer duration. As mentioned earlier, your body stores enough energy for about sixty minutes of serious activity. Glycogen, or stored carbohydrate, needs to be available, but it is stored in limited quantities. However, there is even a better energy source, and that is your fat. If you train the body to utilize fat effectively, then you can continue for longer periods of time because you are tapping into your major energy source. As glycogen is depleted, we must rely more on burning fat for energy and be careful not to reduce glycogen stores too much. So an effective way to build endurance is to exercise in excess of sixty minutes and adapt to using fat better.

Cross-Training

Be careful to not become focused on one activity alone, performing the same routine every day. Runners who are trying to get high numbers of miles covered can easily over train, and actually become slower and over fatigued. A more effective method is referred to as *cross-training*. This is not necessarily the trademarked method called Cross Training, although this can be an effective component of a routine, but simply varying the type of training that you do. Different types of training provide varying benefits, and designing a program that includes periods of different activity can improve overall performance much more effectively. For example, the distance runner would do short sprints, tempo, or pace work for cross-training, as well as incorporate exercises for strength, balance, and stability.

Whenever you change your routine, doing something different becomes another form of challenge, and your body will have to change, or adapt, to keep up with you. The concept of *periodization* utilizes cross-training in spans of time, or cycles. Each cycle is a period of time focused on a specific objective and lasting generally four to six weeks. Each period would include different training routines, often designed to reach a peak of readiness for an athletic or physical event. It is well worth your time to plan out your routine for the entire year. In that year, you create macrocycles and microcycles, in which the exercise plan is changed to emphasize different results. There are times when it is appropriate to just go out and play, but that should be part of the plan.

When you see slower improvements, it may be time to change the routine again. Look at what your overall goal is and plan to advance and peak at the appropriate times. Whenever you change your routine, this is the time when your body makes its greatest changes.

Putting It All Together: Functional Exercise

Why are we building strength and stability, aerobic capacity, and endurance? At some point, we all have to put it together. This is called functional exercise (or, as they called it years ago, sports-specific exercise). Functional exercise is used to rehabilitate and restore the body after injury. But it also really hones our sports-specific skills to a level where we have better coordination and do in fact perform better. It is every bit as important to incorporate different skills and systems into lifelike and sports-like movement. Functional exercise has been developed to do just that.

In functional exercise, you incorporate balance, movement patterns, strength, endurance, and aerobic capacity. The bottom line is that you're putting it all together so that your body can perform as a unit. There are numerous forms of functional exercise, and many different varieties of equipment and devices for its development. Pilates, yoga, various forms of dance, martial arts, boot camps, sports performance, and different forms of exercise training are all forms of functional exercise. You can use balance training apparatus, many assistive devices, kettle balls and lighter weights, and even mats and stability balls. Functional training covers more scope than I can cover in this book.

When you incorporate physical activity into your daily life, you actually start to gain control over the aging process. So many things blamed on aging are actually related to the degeneration that occurs when you don't maintain your body. Exercise is a tool that drives the body to maintain and improve function. You can have a "younger body" through exercise. Physical activity and adaptation creates the body that produces energy, has less stiffness and pain, and actually prevents disease.

Chapter 8

Your New Body

If we only intend to lose weight through burning more calories, it is easy to become unhealthy. If we only do something to alleviate current disease symptoms, like taking vitamin C only when we have a cold, then I believe that we sell ourselves short. When it comes to your health, I don't believe you should plan to just get by. On one hand, you could do like many people and simply breathe enough to just sustain your life. On the other hand, if you take in large, lung-filling breaths and effectively deliver more oxygen to your body, you will have vitality. You can stay alive with a sedentary lifestyle, but your physical abilities won't allow you much freedom. You can stay alive without eating good foods; however, lacking nutrients requires the body to function less effectively.

Consider the fact that even oxygen can easily become a health-limiting nutrient. High blood sugar can impair the red blood cells ability to carry and deliver oxygen. Sleep apnea, where people stop breathing at night, reduces oxygen taken in and delivered. Instead of relying on the CPAP machine for the rest of your life, reduce inflammation, increase the tone in your airways with exercise, and lose some weight. This tends to resolve the apnea. Without good circulation, such as occurs with smoking, oxygen is not delivered. We must pay attention to both structure and function of the body to enjoy wellness.

What I propose is that we consider constructing our physical body so that it performs at a higher level throughout our lifetime. The most common complaint that I hear from people is that they are fatigued. Since one of your most important functions as a living organism is to produce energy, I want you to produce energy efficiently and effectively. Producing more energy will resolve your fatigue. If you ever have a chance to compare the internal structures of a healthy person versus a person who is not, you would see two differently constructed bodies.

In a healthy person, you will find more muscle mass with more and better mitochondria. There is less fat accumulated around the organs producing inflammation. You will find much stronger bones and better tendon and ligament structure, creating strong and stable joints. You will see a large, strong heart that effectively pumps blood throughout the body and large muscular arteries to deliver the blood. A healthy heart can produce eight times the volume of blood with each contraction; therefore the heart does not have to work as hard. You can even see larger, better-myelinated, and better laid-out nerves in a neural network that has been designed, by way of a proper lifestyle, to function so much better.

If we make it our goal to actually construct the best and most efficient human body that we can to live our life in, then we can produce a state of wellness. The important key to this is lifestyle management. If you currently have a healthy body, then keep up your awareness and don't let your body degenerate and "age" too quickly. If you don't have a body that is well constructed, it is never too late to start the remodeling. I encourage you to set today as your first day of regeneration. Any improvement that you can make is going to enhance function.

One of the most important things you will create is referred to as *organ reserve.* When you maintain a state of health, and your biological systems and your internal organs are functioning properly, you tend to compress morbidity into a smaller portion of your lifetime. This ability to minimize disease is what organ reserve is. Proper organ reserve allows you to undergo stress yet remain in balance. If you are healthy and resilient, this indicates that your internal organs are working properly and that they carry a reserve for function. When we get chronically sick, it is a good indication that organ reserve has been lost.

If we use our bodies properly and don't overwhelm them, then we create adaptation and improve the organ reserve. The reason to pursue a lifestyle that creates a better body is to enhance our quality of life and perhaps our longevity. If you sustain an injury and you perform proper rehabilitation, you can often end up with better structure and better function than you had in the first place. Even when you are healthy and you use your mind and your body, you end up with a better neural network, producing improved mental function, coordination, strength, and power.

If you work to remove as much interference as possible, the body will function better. Since I am a chiropractor, I will use chiropractic as one example. Chiropractors automatically practice what is now being referred to as *functional medicine.* Functional medicine deals with how well the body is working and what may be impairing proper function. Instead of identifying a disease and giving it a name, functional medicine looks for patterns of, and solutions to, impaired function. When a chiropractor makes an adjustment in the spine, it is because that doctor has found a part of the spine that is not working as it was designed. If we allow that part of the spine to remain poorly positioned or unable to move freely, we allow interference to the nerves and to the blood vessels around the joint.

By making an "adjustment," the chiropractor restores not only function of a particular joint, but also restores function of the affected systems. The adjustment then tends to reduce pain, improve circulation, enhance nerve transmission, and allow the body to work better and more by design. Anything that is done that removes interference, allowing the body to work better, will enhance health and reduce disease. In functional medicine, the practitioner analyzes patterns and evaluates how best to restore function and reduce dependence on health management. It is better to search for the cause of something and correct the problem at its source.

The right lifestyle coupled with a well-built body is the ultimate goal. That way you stay ahead of the curve and actually live at a biological age that is much lower than the number of years that you've been alive. We do not possess the money or the resources to continue to take care of the people who are sick right now. If we don't do something to change the current situation and its progression, more and more people will be among the sick and need management of chronic disease. If we teach people how to build organ reserve, then we are creating a solution instead of a crisis.

Part Three

Detoxify

Chapter 9

The Case for Detoxification

Every organism has a designed method necessary for getting things in and getting things out. The human body has an entire system for digestion, which brings things in, and then a system for excretion, which transforms things so they can be transported out and then eliminates them. We refer to that excretion system and its associated processes as *detoxification.*

Internally, the body produces toxins through its normal, everyday functions. Biochemical, cellular, and bodily activities generate free radicals and waste products. When these are not handled and eliminated, they can cause irritation to or inflammation of the cells and tissues, blocking normal functions. Fats (especially oxidized fats and oxidized cholesterol), DNA from bacteria and other organisms, and other irritating molecules act as toxins, which can do damage to the body or interfere with its function.

Microbes, including intestinal bacteria, foreign bacteria, yeasts, and parasites, produce metabolic waste products that we must handle in addition to our own waste products. Even the DNA form dead microbes seem to lead to inflammation and the toxic load. Our emotions and stress also generate increased biochemical toxicity. There are several steps in the detoxification process, and as long as it can proceed uninterrupted, the interference is dealt with.

Central to this process is the liver, which can transform many toxic substances into harmless agents and ready them for excretion. While the blood carries waste to the kidneys, the liver also dumps waste through the bile in the intestines, where much of it is eliminated. We also clear toxins when our body sweats. Our sinuses and skin may also be accessory elimination organs, whereby excess mucus or toxins can be released.

If our body is working well, with good immune and eliminative functions, we can handle our basic everyday exposure to toxins. But a problem occurs with excess intake, excess production of toxins, or reduction in the processes of elimination. *Toxicity* occurs in our body when we take in more than what we can utilize and eliminate. Functionally, poor digestion, colon sluggishness and dysfunction, reduced liver function, and poor elimination through the kidneys, respiratory tract, and skin all add to increased toxicity, since things are not being transported out of the body. A toxin may produce an immediate or rapid onset of symptoms, or cause latent, long-term, negative effects. The Reality of Toxicity Living in a chemically-oriented society has made toxicity an ever-increasing concern for the twenty-first century, and the situation grows more perilous each day. The Environmental Protection Agency reports that the average American consumes four pounds of pesticides each year and has residues from over four hundred toxic substances in his or her body. More than three thousand chemical additives are found in the foods we eat. The incidence of many toxic diseases has increased as well, with cancer and cardiovascular disease at the top of the list. Arthritis, allergies, obesity, and many skin problems are other troubles that occur as a result of toxicity. In addition, a wide range of symptoms such as headaches, fatigue, pains, coughs, gastrointestinal problems, and problems from immune dysfunction are all related to toxicity. Toxicity occurs from internal and external sources. We are exposed to toxins daily and can acquire them from our environment by breathing, ingesting, or coming into physical contact with them. Also, most drugs, food additives, and allergens create toxic elements in the body.

Certain things are required to allow the system to work properly. You must consume foods that contain the nutrients required for the detoxification process to be carried out. Eating vegetables is imperative for this, since vegetables contain many of the nutrients and molecules needed to move forward with what is really a process of "biotransformation." Molecules are changed chemically, or transformed, so that they may be eliminated. Vegetables are also a good source of fiber, which is important in the cleaning and clearing of toxic and excess substances. If you don't consume enough vegetables and some fruits, then the system will be impaired, since it does not have the raw materials and substances necessary to proceed. You also must drink plenty of clean water, since the process of biotransformation converts dangerous molecules to something water soluble. Without proper hydration, your system cannot work toward, and fulfill, elimination.

In fact, one of the most important things you can do to facilitate detoxification is to exercise. You cannot simply depend on the heart to pump all of the fluids in your body through blood vessels and the lymphatic system. To transport and process toxins, you need blood and lymph to travel full circuit. Good circulation is paramount to accomplish this and to cleanse the body. First of all, exercise is necessary for these fluids that transport the toxins to move through their systems effectively. Without the action of muscles and a strong pump (your heart), the detoxification system can be left at a literal standstill. Many systems, such as energy production, are completely dependent on physical activity levels. Your elimination system requires a great deal of energy to proceed normally. If you are not physically active, the systems will not effectively operate, and you will be in stasis. Stasis means no appreciable movement of fluids and no processing, which means no transformation or elimination of substances that are interfering with function.

Medical toxicologists tend to think in terms of a single toxin and its isolated effects. They tend to think in absolute values applying to everyone. Substances are graded at levels where there is no observed adverse effect (NOAEL), or often in terms of how much of a single substance it takes to create a problem. There is also the lowest observed adverse effect level (LOAEL). In this case, scientists will refer to the "maximum tolerable concentration" or "maximum tolerable dose" of something. A substance might also have a minimum lethal concentration or minimum lethal dose, and a median lethal concentration or median lethal dose. (The substance concentration in the body that is enough to kill 50 percent of the people is commonly called the LD 50.) Finally, there is the absolute concentration or dose, or the amount of a substance that will kill everyone.

These criteria are commonly used to determine if something can be regarded as safe for you to consume, or even to use as a chemical product. Limits of exposure are based on these established levels. The only problem with this system is that our bodies do not live in isolation, with one exposure at a time. In your lifetime—or for that matter, in any given span of time—you are exposed to many different things, sometimes all at once. Some substances by themselves will have no ill effect, but mixed with the right second or third substance, they will become immediately lethal. A more meaningful measurement is the ***total body burden,*** which is the cumulative effect of one substance after another building up until the body can no longer handle it, which is when we start seeing symptoms of disease and physical damage. Only recently has the total body burden been seriously considered in conjunction with new exposures to measure risk.

Over time, without proper cleansing and elimination, your body will inevitably accumulate a number of various harmful substances. The human body really only has two paths to take. The body can either chemically transform and then eliminate these substances, or the body can store them away primarily in fatty tissues. One possible repository is your accumulated fat stores; another is your brain. The better scenario is to transfer these substances to the outside. The body must deal with its own physiological waste products and metabolites, in addition to heavy metals, persistent organic pollutants, parasites, bacteria, viruses, and even the prescription medication that you introduce into your body.

A major source of these toxins is actually the food that you eat every day. Today there are so many substances added to food that modify or alter or block our biological systems. Your foods contain all sorts of new ingredients, such as preservatives, emulsifiers, flavor enhancers, food coloring, fillers, and even altered proteins from genetically modified foods. These things cause a level of interference or alteration in how your body works. If your body cannot function as designed or evolved to function, then you will have deal with the modern chronic diseases that occur from dysfunction. That is why whenever I've had somebody do a cleanse (see chapter 11), we see an improvement in their clinical symptoms.

When people are overwhelmed with toxins, that total body burden not only interrupts function but begins to create physical damage. Many neurodevelopmental and neurologic disorders are the result of toxicity. Some toxins do not allow nerve tissue to develop; other toxins damage existing nerve tissue. Toxins like mercury actually demyelinate existing nerves and can create a situation much like multiple sclerosis. And your toxic body burden can impair the entire process of memory, learning, and focus, specifically the process of neural cell growth and the myelination of nerves.

Immune system toxicity impairs the body's ability to respond when needed to threats foreign substances create. At the same time, this toxicity of the immune system creates a situation where the immune system becomes hyper-reactive. The term used is called *hypersensitivity*, which is really a measure of your environmental tolerance. When you have a large body burden and substances themselves are triggering more immune response, the body becomes too quick to react to almost anything else, and tolerance is lost. This is in essence what an allergy is: little or no tolerance even to things natural in the environment. The good news is that as you reduce the body burden, the allergy symptoms improve, because the body is now more tolerant. This even has a positive impact on problems such as multiple chemical sensitivity.

Realize that toxicity affects your metabolism and, more importantly, the mitochondria. Remember that mitochondria are your fuel cells. The mitochondrion is where your energy is created, and without energy, nothing can function. Take the batteries out of your favorite toy, and no matter how many times you flip the on/off switch, nothing will happen. If you lose enough and damage enough of your mitochondria, you may as well have taken your own batteries (fuel cells) out.

Many researchers have concluded that perhaps the most important function of the human body is the production of energy. If you can't produce enough energy, then in a sense, your health and perhaps your life are compromised. Yet one of the most sensitive systems to toxins, and even to drugs like antibiotics, is your energy production system. Mitochondria are easily interfered with, damaged, and even destroyed. Substances that interfere with the mitochondria are also interfering with the body's ability to produce the energy required. When you're fatigued, the problem is really that you cannot provide enough energy to run all of your systems. The complication is when energy production is experiencing interference to such an extent that you are too fatigued to even produce enough energy to detoxify and remove the interference. If you cannot produce enough energy to clear out substances that interfere with energy production itself, this can become a very serious situation.

In the fast-growing area of study on the effects of toxicity, science is also demonstrating a great deal of hormone disruption. We now know more about all the plastics, chemicals, and everything that interferes with or can mimic the body's hormones. Hormones must be in balance, must be able to interact with their specific receptors, and must be properly disposed of, or they become toxins themselves. Many of the chemicals that we eat directly in food, or package our food with, end up getting into our bodies and causing hormone disruption.

These chemicals change the internal environment and therefore also change the function of hormones and even genetic expression. When hormones themselves are not metabolized correctly, many of the metabolites themselves cause dysfunction and damage to the body. This is one of the biggest dangers for women using hormones such as Premarin. The conjugated equine estrogens are different from human estrogens and are higher in number. When the body goes to metabolize, or break down, these foreign estrogens, they are broken down into some dangerous byproducts that themselves do harm.

Another new area of study is called genotoxicity, which is the actual change to and disruption of how DNA functions and the shortening of the DNA itself. Toxins that alter and damage DNA drastically change the way that your body functions and restores itself. The ultimate disruption often shows up in the creation of cancer and other serious diseases, because DNA cannot be referenced accurately. Even more disturbing is the effect of mutation or change in the DNA. This is like rewriting the playbook for your body. The consequences can be huge.

Several studies have been done on the body burden of newborn babies. It was assumed in the past that infants were pretty safe since they had not been exposed very long to the environment. A group called the Environmental Working Group (www.ewg.org) did a study on newborn umbilical-cord blood and found that the babies at birth had already been well dosed with chemicals delivered by their mother. On average, there was evidence of two hundred chemicals being delivered to the babies.

Your brain and other major organs are directly affected by your total body burden. Most commonly, toxins in the body are recognized and then trigger an immune response. When these toxins are present all the time, so are the immune-mediating molecules that keep your body in a high state of inflammation. So not only do the toxins themselves cause damage and dysfunction, but they are able to trigger and prolong an inflammatory response. We know that many brain disorders turn out to be the result of ongoing inflammation. The extreme case of an inflammatory response is when your own immune system begins to attack your tissues. We refer to this as autoimmune disease, and it is much more prevalent today than ever before.

If you notice symptoms of unexplained fatigue, sluggish elimination, irritated skin, airborne allergies or food allergies, low-grade infections, bags under your eyes, a distended stomach even if the rest of your body is thin, menstrual difficulties, skin problems, and even mental confusion, this is reliable evidence that your body is already overwhelmed. These symptoms are evidence that your body has accumulated more toxins than it is eliminating. This accumulation is your total body burden. When the total body burden interferes with the function of the human body, dysfunction occurs, and symptoms are the result of dysfunction. Many symptoms and diseases tend to disappear if this burden is reduced.

How Can We Improve Detoxification? You make a choice with every mouthful of food and with every pill that you take. You have the power to choose whether or not many of these toxins get into your body in the first place. Foods are adulterated to give them better shelf life, better appearance or consistency, and even to stimulate you to want more. *Excitotoxins* is a term used by many neurologists, such as Dr. David Perlmutter and Dr. Russell Blaylock, to name a few. What they are referring to are chemicals intentionally placed in food to enhance their taste or to stimulate your hunger or thirst. In the past, substances like salt or sugar were used to keep you wanting more. Bars and restaurants would add salt to food so that people would drink more beer and consume more food. Now we have "better living through chemistry" and a number of modern-day chemicals. Monosodium glutamate or MSG, aspartate, and other chemicals are added to food and act as enhancers or nerve exciters. However, if excited in excess, the nerves actually become damaged, so that physical and mental problems are initiated.

Unfortunately, it is your responsibility to be aware of the amount of toxic burden that you introduce into your body. You cannot depend on the government to make the right decision for you. One very effective strategy is to simply eat real food instead of food that is altered or adulterated. You could reduce or eliminate items like coffee and alcohol. Both of these have actually demonstrated health benefits if used appropriately, but they can also produce not-so-healthy side effects. Caffeine, alcohol, and other substances have to be detoxified. They are run through the same system and hopefully eliminated. A common test for liver function utilizes caffeine and aspirin and measures how well they are metabolized. In defense of coffee, we sometimes use it to induce or start the detoxification process, and it has benefits since it contains antioxidants.

I would suggest that you eliminate cigarettes, since they negatively affect the chemical environment of your body. Cigarette smoking damages circulation, changes pH (acidity), and alters normal chemistry, while directly damaging tissue. Reduce your intake of refined sugars, realizing that sugar is a toxin itself. Do not consume altered fats, such as partially hydrogenated fat; remove it completely from your dietary intake. Many other items are toxic and set up a toxic environment. Minimize the use of chemical-based household cleaners and personal healthcare products. It does make a difference when you use natural alternatives.

A seven-day juice fast can be productive if you're drinking fresh fruit and vegetable juices. If not designed correctly, though, there will be too high a concentration of sugar, some phytonutrients, a lack of intact fiber and even processing chemicals. I may use a juice fast with conditions such as cancer, where I want a high dose of plant nutrients.

There are cleansing supplement packages that contain fiber, vitamins, herbs, minerals, and protein together to make the cleanse a "supportive cleanse." Also, there are functional foods specifically designed for certain physical conditions, and these can be effectively used while cleansing. Sometimes I will utilize one of these predesigned foods with one green vegetable each day for a week with great results. There are a few products that we use specifically for diabetics and for inflammatory bowel diseases that we've gotten great results with using this way.

A cleanse does not have to be complicated; it can be as simple as a diet consisting of only real food. It is good to eliminate commonly known allergens, so I suggest that the diet is gluten free, dairy free, citrus free, nut free, egg free, and perhaps free of other foods like corn or even soy. That still leaves you with quite a choice of foods and less chance of a physical response.

I actually prefer that most people do a cleanse lasting around twenty-eight days. With this plan, the body has the time to accomplish the collection, biotransformation, and elimination of the toxins. Fasting or liquid diets for two to five days, followed by a carefully planned elimination diet, can be very effective, since you are resting the systems.

Supplements, herbs, exercise, dry skin brushing, and hydrotherapy can enhance circulation and the entire detoxification effect. One example of hydrotherapy would be to take a very hot shower for five minutes, and then follow with cold water for thirty seconds. Do this three times, and then lie down for thirty minutes.

Sweating, especially in a dry sauna, is a very good way to eliminate waste products. For some chemicals, it may be literally the only way to remove them. Exercise is effective for sweating; however, in exercise, blood is moving in toward the muscles as well as to the skin surface for cooling. In a dry sauna, more blood is sent out to the surface for cooling, and toxins will then be picked up at a greater rate to be excreted to sweat glands.

I cannot overstate the importance of exercise. The enhancement to circulation and the whole detoxification system cannot be matched. Remember that exercise has the ability to restore function by actually turning systems back on. When you exercise, you increase the production of energy and enhance the efficiency of anything that the body does.

Fiber including brown rice, organically grown vegetables, and fresh fruits are excellent detoxifying foods. Fiber can absorb toxins, clean the intestine, and then is eliminated along with the toxins. Beets, radishes, artichokes, cabbage, broccoli, spirulina, Chorella, and seaweed are good choices to incorporate during a cleanse. Herbs such as milk thistle, green tea, dandelion root, and burdock root actively induce detoxification and cleansing while they also protect the liver. Vitamin C and cysteine help in the production of glutathione, which is a great antioxidant as well as a molecule used in detoxification.

Again, it is very important to be hydrated, and we recommend drinking half of your body weight (pounds) in ounces of water. Breathing, if done properly, will allow more oxygen to circulate, is an effective route for elimination of toxins, has a wonderful ability to reduce the effects of stress.

I see many cases where a detoxification strategy has completely reversed or resolved serious physical conditions. Instead of relying on prescription after prescription of more chemicals, it turns out to be a much better plan to remove chemicals that are already there and resolve the problem that way.

The whole strategy here is to build a condition of optimal function and optimal health—or, in other words, build organ reserve. Dr. James Fries, the first to propose this concept, stated that a patient needed good "organ reserve" to compress morbidity or sickness to the smallest part of his or her lifetime. Organ reserve is the resiliency you have toward avoiding disease, and this reserve will fluctuate depending on how you live your life. A major way to improve organ reserve is to remove interference to function and let the organs rest and recover.

Your toxic burden might be described as an unflushed toilet. I encourage you to flush that toilet, to cleanse, and send the waste for processing by eliminating it from your house (your body). If you don't, it's called constipation. While you are constipated, you are reabsorbing some of the toxins that your body worked very hard to process for elimination. Many people live with this toxic burden and even add to it. When the burden reaches a certain threshold, they begin have symptoms. This still may not be enough to get them concerned. When those symptoms proceed into diseases, that is the point that most people act. It would have been so much simpler to simply flush the toilet and not deal with the final result.

Your body works very hard to eliminate heavy metals, persistent organic pollutants, biological organisms (viral, bacterial, fungal, and parasites), and your own physiological waste products. The detoxification system is functionally dependent on gut and liver health, hormone balance, and nutritional status.

Detoxification is a very natural process that is designed to clean the blood and the body tissues. When we plan or structure a cleanse in our clinic, what we want to do is support or induce this process of elimination. For your health, you need to remove impurities from the blood, and this is done to a great degree inside your liver. The liver is where many toxins are processed to facilitate elimination. The body eliminates toxins through the kidneys, intestines, lungs, lymph, and skin. When the system is compromised and impurities are not properly filtered and transformed, the entire body will be affected adversely.

A formal detoxification or cleansing program can help the body's natural cleaning process by allowing a period of rest for all of your internal organs. There are also things that can be done to stimulate the liver or induce it toward transforming these toxins into something that can be eliminated rather than stored. The next step is to promote or facilitate the elimination of substances through the intestines, kidneys, skin, and even your lungs. Anything that can be done to improve circulation of both blood and lymph, such as physical activity, really contributes to the effectiveness of the system. Perhaps more important than anything is providing the necessary nutrients and being able to efficiently generate the energy required for the process to continue.

I recommend patients do some form of detoxification at least once a year. A good program is generally safe and beneficial to your health. If, while doing a cleanse, you really struggle with symptoms, it is quite possible that you are doing too much and proceeding too fast. One common situation is called the Hertzheimer reaction. This reaction occurs as toxic substances within the body are released after being inert and stored away. To some extent, when people are doing a formal detoxification program, there may be symptoms produced, but the cleansing process is not designed to make you sick. Cleansing requires some effort, but it may have to be interrupted and modified if you experience such strong reactions. It is important to pay attention to how you are progressing while doing a cleanse.

If you grow your own food, drink only clean water, exercise regularly, and live out away from environmental pollutants, then you probably don't have to undergo regular detoxification protocols. However, if you're like most people—living in the city, consuming foods designed for convenience, not physically active, not having regular bowel movements, and suffering daily exposure to various pollutants—then you would benefit from cleansing on a periodic basis. You can find our basic cleansing protocol in chapter 11.

Chapter 10

You Can't Judge a Book by Its Cover

The Healthy Suspicion of Food Labels

The most effective way to reduce the total body burden would be to keep undesirable substances and molecules out of the body in the first place. By far, the greatest source of both nutrients and toxic substances is through your mouth. By this route you expose your digestive tract to many things in the environment that would be better kept outside. People are much too trusting when it comes to the purchase of foods and household chemicals, as well as personal care products. Anything that requires a label should immediately come under scrutiny. If it is going to get into your mouth, or on your skin, or inhaled, I want to know what is in it.

Wholesome, original foods don't need a label. If you eat real foods, there is much less need to police ingredients for safety, search for nutrients, or even count calories. Once the industrial process of packaging and processing begins, ensure your safety. Just because it is on the shelf and available in the store, does not mean that it is safe to use or is in any way good for you. Yes, there are laws and standards, but the government cannot protect you from every exposure, and sometimes the government is causing the exposure. It is for you to learn and decide if something is safe, or if it is not. Real foods, like an apple, are recognized without a label, and with the exception of knowledge about pesticide use or perhaps genetic modification, if the food is organic, we are better off.

Everything else is a judgment call, and the place to start is the required label. You cannot judge a food by its marketing, either by the printed pictures or the health claims. It is of ultimate importance that you pay attention to the ingredients and things listed in the label, which you will put into or on your own body. Of course, I would ask you to pay attention to the environment in which you live, and to things that you are exposed to from the outside world. Every route of entry is to be considered. But many scientists regard your digestive tract as still being in contact with the outside of your body. What you choose to eat—the things that you put into your own mouth—need to have careful consideration.

Remember, food is a form of communication to your body from the outside world. There is an entirely new science referred to as xenohormesis, which has to do with this communication from outside of ourselves. *Xeno* means foreign to the body, or from the environment outside, and *hormesis* is when a small amount of something has a much larger than expected effect, denoting some form of communication. The nutrients and chemicals that plants produce, once introduced into the human body, can generate such an effect and response. It has actually been demonstrated that plants communicate to us, telling us about the conditions in our environment. If the plant is stressed by something like a drought, it will produce certain stress chemicals in response. Our body, upon consuming the plant, mounts a response as well based on that information. The plant literally communicates with us, as do other real foods.

If you are consuming food like substances, or processed foods, not only is this communication broken, but other communication, inaccurate in content, is established. By eating things that are not true food, like most commercially processed foods, you will get a communicated effect, but not the one you're looking for. Small amounts of toxic substances will have their effect as the body responds and tries to deal with their breakdown and elimination. It does not take very much of many toxic substances to hurt you or even kill you.

Take a walk through the average supermarket, and especially in the center of the market you will find things so foreign that they have to be labeled as edible, or as food. You wouldn't really know that they were food otherwise. If you routinely consume processed and adulterated substances, even if they may have started out as a food (for example, a bread or cereal product), then you not only will be lacking in nutrients and beneficial substances, but you increase exposure to things that are toxic. A toxic substance can do damage by itself, or it can communicate or induce a process to a body and then induce symptoms in reaction.

Even in a health food store you cannot simply trust that everything on the shelf is good for you. Please be careful to make good judgments on everything. If you're unsure, then just don't eat it. Many things that are approved for sale and sitting on the shelf are not necessarily even fit for you to consume at all. If you are eating something on a regular basis that is no longer identifiable as food, then is it worth considering making a change to your favorite snack?

You have been led to believe that the FDA and the USDA serve and protect the public's health. Yet there are many known conflicts of interest between these and other government agencies and industries. Pharmaceutical and industrial food corporations have a lot of influence and have monopolized access to the drug and food approval process. Over 100,000 people are killed and over 2 million injured per year by legally prescribed drugs. Two thirds of the FDA's own scientists do not believe the agency can adequately monitor the safety of drugs. Many of those on the approval boards also work for those companies that are submitting drugs for approval.

The system is somewhat broken, and I am bringing this up to encourage you to investigate everything that you eat, everything that you use in personal care, and even the prescribed medications that you take. What are you using the product for or even taking the drug for? What are the expected effects and what are the benefits? What are the possible negative effects that may occur? Monitor closely if the medication or product is helping and is doing what was expected. As we mentioned in a previous chapter, with prescription medication, how long will you be required to take the medication, and what will be the strategy to discontinue its use as soon as possible? There are only a few drugs that require a lifetime of use. Most medications produced are studied for short-term use only, and most medications will not be necessary when you restore function to your own body.

It is also well worth your time to know more about the products that you use in your day-to-day life. Some of the products in your home right now could have potentially devastating effects. Many personal care products, cleaning products, and things that you use from day to day are better utilized if you know their potential for harm. Consider that even many air fresheners contain chemicals that we now know to be dangerous to human beings. More and more is being learned about plastics and other chemicals in our environment that produce health consequences.

Please read any label and take the necessary precautions printed there. Even though there are labeling laws and regulations in effect, it seems the majority of people do not even bother to read them. The warnings are there for a reason, and we all need to pay closer attention. It's amazing how many people suffer injury that could have been avoided by simply paying attention to the precautions on a label. If you start reading the labels, you will likely be surprised at how much unnatural chemistry you may be introducing into your own body.

Numerous surveys have been done with people to see if they could actually interpret something as simple as a food label. Generally, more than half the people cannot actually figure the labels out. One of the most commonly missed factors is the serving size. It is a common mistake for people not to multiply the amounts on the label to match the number of servings they will actually consume. If you read the ingredient listings, this is an indication of relative concentrations, since ingredients are listed in order of amount in that food. In other words, the first item in the list is present in higher amount than the next item, and this continues in order of concentration.

If sugar is listed first, I recommend you put that item back on the shelf. If there are a number of unnatural chemicals, I also recommend that you put the item back. Yet millions of people consume pounds and pounds of substances that are actually dangerous to the human body. I further recommend that you start frequenting farmers markets, or even buying straight from the farm. This can be done in many areas of the country, and some farm products can be shipped direct to consumer. If you shop at a supermarket frequently, then take Dr. Barry Sears' advice and avoid the center of the market. Most markets are designed in a way that you will find the healthier foods on the perimeter.

Since we are discussing judgments about food and things that are food like, let's discuss judgments based on food packaging and marketing. Children do not choose cereals and other things to eat based on their nutritional value; they choose cereals based on the character pictured on the front or the toy contained inside. We have to be careful not to fall into the same trap. It is easy to make a quick judgment on something based on pictures and buzzwords. If you rely on claims printed on the package, you may be surprised when you get the package home to find that it was not wholesome food. I have actually purchased something that I thought was wholesome and organic, only to find out that it was highly processed and adulterated. It is important to determine if what is inside the package is made for the human body and will promote health. Most processed foods present the body with difficulties.

Just because you see a quaint little farm or a smiling farmer pictured on the package does not mean this is a representation of where this food came from. Is the food you're buying to consume organic? Does it contain pesticides, preservatives, or growth factors? Was it genetically modified or altered in some way? How much has been done to it between its harvest and your table? Your body has evolved to utilize certain original foods; everything else presents a new challenge, and sometimes an overwhelming challenge. That overwhelming challenge leads down the path to disease.

Unfortunately, we cannot depend on the endorsements given by certain associations and societies. These are paid endorsements, and many times the food endorsed has no relationship to the supposed study that allowed endorsement. We have to investigate for ourselves to find the truth. The media will have you believe that if you take that pill, drink that drink, or eat that food, then you will have happiness and health. Just be careful who you believe and what their motives are. Don't buy something simply because one of your favorite celebrities endorses it. Look into what it is and whether or not it will really benefit you.

Good Things to Look for on the Label

So let's consider some of the information that you can find on a food label. First of all, as we mentioned earlier, consider the serving size and ensure that you are calculating ingredient amounts based on how much you will actually consume. The nutrition facts will give a serving size and then the amount per serving. You want to consider the number of calories from carbohydrates and then determine the net carbohydrates. To do this, take the total number and subtract fiber, sugar alcohols, non-sugar sweeteners, and any other carbohydrate that will not impact blood sugar levels. Now you have a better idea of that food's impact on your blood sugar and ultimately on your health. A lower glycemic index food will also show less net carbohydrates.

Consider the amount of protein, the source of that protein, and how much the protein has been altered. If you consume animal products, see if you can determine if the animal was healthy. Beef and other red meat will ideally be from grass-fed stock. When the animal consumes its natural diet, it will be healthier. That translates to healthier food for you. If you do not consume animal products, it is still important to consider the sources of your protein. If it is an extracted or processed protein product, then how was it processed? It is very important that if you utilize a whey, hemp, pea, or other protein supplement that the protein is unaltered from natural protein. Heat, genetic modification, and pressure can all alter the protein until it is no longer real food. The best protein supplements are cold processed and packaged safely. Even the consumption of dairy products will vary in safety. There are many people who can tolerate organic and raw dairy products but are reactive to the processed "dairy foods" you find in stores.

What is the fat content of the food you're about to buy? What are the types of fat that it contains, and is the fat safe to consume and beneficial to you as a natural good fat? If you see a list of colorings, flavorings, enhancements, hormones, and perhaps even pesticides, it is better to just put that food back on the shelf. There are also many fillers, binders, and extenders added to your food. Although these are generally regarded as safe to consume, they really have no benefit for you. Some things are added in order to get more out of a smaller source of food. You've probably done this at home, say, in making meatloaf. You're able to take a small amount of meat and add grain, and suddenly it seemed as if you had more meat. Many people consume a lot of cellulose from trees, which is legally added to food. This is done sometimes to change the food's characteristics, and other times just to make more product to sell.

Labeling nutritional facts also requires the labeling of the recommended daily allowance (RDA) or dietary reference intake (DRI). These measure what percentage of the total recommended daily amount of recognized nutrients is in each serving based on a 2,000-calorie diet. These daily values are for adults and children four years of age or over. These values are established by the government and indicate a recommended nutrient intake. These recommended daily amounts are often based on avoiding a deficiency disease. For example, if you don't receive generally about 30 milligrams of vitamin C each day, then you will create a deficiency disease called scurvy. Most if not all nutrients, when at a low-enough level, will lead to a certain type of disease or physical condition.

Protein deficiency can lead to kwashiorkor, marasmus, and mental or emotional problems. Kwashiorkor is typically seen when a child is weaned from high-protein breast milk to start eating a diet primarily of processed carbohydrates. The common presentation is a swollen belly due to edema, as well as weakness, poor growth, and a much higher susceptibility to diseases. This disease can also occur in adults with eating disorders or when hospitalized and not receiving sufficient protein intake. These people tend to lose a lot of muscle and organ tissue, literally wasting away. PEM, or protein energy malnutrition, can result in reduced brain functioning, reduced brain growth and repair, and nerve damage.

However, it is more common that people do not consume enough quality protein, or they experience difficulties in digesting proteins, creating a deficiency of amino acids. We often test amino acid levels in blood (or sometimes urine), finding deficiencies and imbalances in specific amino acids. The treatment includes giving these patients certain amino acids in their free form and improving their digestive capabilities. This can be a lifesaver for people with mental and emotional disorders, as well as for those with physical dysfunctions. In the past, it was assumed that Americans consumed so much protein that protein deficiency should not be of concern. However, with the rampant use of proton pump inhibitors given to people with indigestion, I find many people become protein deficient, since without the acid in the stomach, they do not properly digest the poor proteins they do consume.

In most circumstances, there is no absolute dietary requirement for carbohydrates. Certain cells utilize carbohydrates, requiring glucose as a fuel. But most cells can also run on ketones, the breakdown products of fat) as well as protein, which is converted to carbohydrates. Our bodies have been designed such that we can do very well with ketones. In fact, a very effective treatment for nerve function and seizure disorders is called a protein-sparing modified fast. This is a very low carbohydrate intake designed to put the body into ketosis (less than 50g). This is not the same as ketoacidosis, which is dangerous in diabetes.

In fact, ketogenic diets look very promising in the treatment of cancer, since the cancer cells need sugar and cannot survive on ketones. This is not to say that we all need to avoid carbohydrates. Reasonable carbohydrate intake is effective at enhancing performance, and certain forms of carbohydrate do have great benefit and are utilized well by the body. It is certain carbohydrates in excess that we need to be wary of.

Essential fatty acids are termed essential for a reason. There is a real need for good fats in the diet. Deficiency tends to include dry skin, hair loss, impaired wound healing, and malfunctioning throughout the nervous system, including the brain. Without these fats, the brain and the entire neural network cannot restore itself or function correctly. The whole process of learning is based on the process of myelination of nerves. Without essential fats, cells don't function, nerves don't build myelin, hormones become deficient, and neurotransmitters can't function. For more on this, refer back to our macronutrient discussion.

A deficiency of vitamin A is related to night blindness, or difficulty seeing in dim light. A deficiency of this vitamin will also create a number of skin conditions, problems with taste and smell, and even causes difficulty with reproductive capacity. In addition to these things, vitamin A is an important player in the integrity and function of your immune system.

Vitamin B_1 (thiamine) deficiency produces beriberi. This disease can cause an accumulation of fluid throughout the body and even lead to sudden death. In dry beriberi, there is paralysis and polyneuritis. In cases of alcoholism and poor diet, a condition called Wernicke–Korsakoff syndrome can be manifested, causing rapid eye movements loss of muscle coordination mental confusion and memory loss. Food sources for this vitamin are meats, wheat germ, whole grains, and legumes like nuts and beans.

Vitamin B_2 (riboflavin) deficiency is known as ariboflavinosis. Symptoms include cracks in the skin at the corner of the mouth, fissures of the lips, and an inflamed, magenta-colored tongue. Milk products and cereals are sources of vitamin B_2.

Vitamin B_3 (niacin) deficiency creates symptoms of diarrhea, dermatitis, and dementia. If the disease remains untreated, it can also lead to death. This is commonly called pellagra. It is interesting that corn will deplete niacin and lead to pellagra, because corn is so low in the amino acid tryptophan, which can lead to a B_3 deficiency. In extreme cases, niacin deficiency even leads to schizophrenia. Historically, this has happened in the American corn belt where a large number of cases of schizophrenia developed and were subsequently cured with the administration of niacin. In fact, there is an entire science of orthomolecular psychiatry initiated by Dr. Abram Hoffer, an MD psychiatrist who effectively treated schizophrenia and other mental disorders using high doses of niacin and other nutrients.

Vitamin B_6 (pyridoxine) is essential for the metabolism of protein, the synthesis of neurotransmitters, and other critical functions in the body. Deficiency leads to dermatitis, microcytic hypochromic anemia, impaired immune function, depression, confusion, and convulsions. Several medications interfere with B_6. As a supplement, it is best taken in the form called P5P.

Vitamin B_5 (pantothenic acid) deficiency can cause fatigue, irritability, sleep disturbances, abdominal distress, and neurological disorders such as numbness in the hands and feet.

Biotin is known for enhancing nails, hair, and skin. Deficiency can lead to skin rashes, hair loss, and even neurological abnormalities.

Folate, sometimes referred to as vitamin B_9 works closely along with vitamin B_{12}. These vitamins participate in DNA synthesis. Deficiency leads to weakness and fatigue from megaloblastic anemia. Deficiency of folate causes disruption of cell division in the gastrointestinal tract, resulting in persistent diarrhea and impaired synthesis of white blood cells and platelets. An inadequate intake in early pregnancy may cause neural tube defects in the fetus.

Vitamin B_{12} (cobalamin) deficiency can also result in megaloblastic anemia. Vitamin B_{12} maintains the myelin sheath that protects nerve fibers, and its deficiency leads to nerve degeneration, from numbness to eventually paralysis. It is also important cofactor in metabolic processes. It is commonly purchased as cyanocobalamin but some people must be careful, even though it is just a small amount of cyanide. I prefer to utilize methylcobamin.

Vitamin C (ascorbic acid) deficiency produces scurvy. It is also known to be potentiated, or more effective, when taken with certain bioflavonoids that occur normally in foods. Scurvy can cause hemorrhaging of tissues, leaving bruises under the skin and swollen gums that usually become infected. The membranes of the heart and brain are affected and damaged. Wounds heal slowly and the bleeding around internal organs can be fatal.

There is also the lack of effective collagen production. The disease is slow to develop and is manifested early by fatigue, irritability, and depression. Even a slight deficiency of vitamin C can be responsible for acne, easy bruising, sore gums, and hemorrhaging around bones. Sources of vitamin C are citrus fruit, broccoli, strawberries, kiwi, cantaloupe, and many other fruits and vegetables. Vitamin C is probably best known for its ability to shorten the duration of colds and flu.

Calcium deficiency can be responsible for osteoporosis, rickets, and tetany.

Vitamin D deficiency is known to cause a bone disease called rickets. It was common to infants and children until the introduction of vitamin D–enriched foods. Your bones require sufficient various minerals, but they need the vitamin D for modeling. In rickets, the bones become soft and deformed, and there is rheumatic pain. More recently though, vitamin D, which is really a seco hormone has been studied further and found to be a very important hormonal substance in the body. It has been shown to be a very potent antiviral as well as a stimulator of immune response in other pathways.

Vitamin D also interacts with a large number of your genes and is responsible for many processes working smoothly and even initiating some of them. It also has a close relationship with the thyroid gland and other hormones. The most efficient source of vitamin D is UVB or sun exposure. Interestingly, vitamin D works to prevent skin cancer. There are fortified foods, but they tend to contain vitamin D_2. I recommend that you have your serum level tested for the 25–OH form of D and supplement with vitamin D_3 if levels are below 50 ng/mL.

Vitamin E deficiency can lead to hemolysis, neuromuscular dysfunction that causes a loss of reflex, impaired balance and coordination, and muscle weakness and visual disturbances. It is also an important antioxidant protecting cells and tissues from free-radical attack.

Vitamin K is necessary for the formation of blood-clotting factors and also plays a part in bone metabolism. Its deficiency can lead to impaired clotting of the blood and internal bleeding, even without trauma.

Iodine deficiency will interfere with thyroid function and can lead to goiter or enlargement of the thyroid.

Iron deficiency leads to anemia of the blood, since iron is needed for red blood cell production.

Potassium deficiency includes weakness, loss of appetite, muscle cramping, and confusion. Severe deficiency may result in a cardiac arrhythmia.

Selenium deficiency can lead to Keshan disease, a cardiomyopathy. Selenium is also very important in combating viral infection and is necessary for the proper function of the thyroid.

Zinc deficiency can lead to growth retardation. It is also important for tissue healing and fertility. It is the constituent of numerous enzymes and regulates gene expression.

All nutrients work together with, and in ratios to, each other. In many cases, it is not a simple deficiency but truly an imbalance created between nutrients. In fact, there is no way to determine exactly how much of a certain nutrient that your body will require each day. Your best and most effective strategy is to consume real food that is nutrient rich so that your body has an ongoing supply. If you are eating processed food with a label, look for nutrient density and quality.

There is a big difference between simply sustaining life and having a body in optimal health. If you begin to shut down or impair the biological systems that make up your body, then you have started to experience dysfunction. Dysfunction starts exhibiting itself as symptoms and eventually builds into an entire disease process. Feeding your body the nutrients that it requires from food delivers nutrients in their best form, with all the supporting nutrients in place. Eating labeled foods will more likely require supplementation. In fact, some of the best supplements are real-food concentrates. Eat the more commonly consumed diet of flour products and processed foods that tend to be lacking in nutrient density, and you force your body to triage.

In current research, there are only two ways that are proven to directly impact longevity, health, and vitality. One is exercise. Physical activity above a certain level of intensity requires the body to adapt and retain or improve healthy function, as we have discussed. The second effective impact on your health, now proven scientifically, is referred to as caloric restriction. I am not talking about fasting or the absence of calories altogether. This is about consuming nutrient-dense foods, which creates a lower calorie intake. The effect of the consumption of fewer calories is prevalent in research, demonstrating a positive effect on everything from dementia, Alzheimer's, and cognitive function to weight control and overall proper function of the human body. We can't seem to handle the excess of calories abundant in labeled foods. We can handle eating an abundance of real food.

Let's finish this chapter with an example of requirements for nutrient intake. Dr. Linus Pauling, a well-published researcher, double Nobel Prize winner, and an inventor, had a keen interest in vitamin C. In his research on vitamin C, he found that in the animals that can produce this nutrient, there was a two-hundred-fold difference in vitamin C production from day to day. Some days the animal had a need for a small amount, and on other days more was produced to meet a higher demand. Human beings cannot produce their own vitamin C; it has to be introduced into the body through food or supplements. How much should you take? Well, Dr. Pauling wondered that as well. When he studied animals again who could make vitamin C, and then related those animals to human beings, adjusting for size and other parameters, he found that human beings probably required about 9,000 milligrams per day for health. It only takes about 30 milligrams per day to avoid scurvy.

In fact, Dr. Pauling was known to take as much as 18,000 mg when he thought he might get a cold. He and others believe this is part of what kept him healthy into his nineties. In our clinic, we would give doses of 50,000 to 100,000 milligrams by IV. Some people claim that vitamin C is toxic at certain levels. I have not seen any good research demonstrating this, and we saw no detrimental effect while administering high doses. High-dose vitamin C looks promising even for cancer treatment. It is a nutrient the body seems to do very well with, the common side effect being bowel tolerance. Bowel tolerance will change, with the body in general getting used to higher dosages of ascorbic acid, but in the beginning at a certain oral dose there may be gas, bloating, and diarrhea.

So, how much vitamin C do we need? No one really knows the amount. Some very good science indicates that around 2,000 milligrams to 3,000 milligrams or above is a good place to start. The RDA was only based on not developing deficiency disease, or scurvy. Knowing that 30 milligrams would prevent scurvy, the government put in a safety factor and came up with an RDA of up to 60 milligrams per day. The DRI goes as high as 120 milligrams recommended, with an upper limit of 200 per day. Again, Dr. Pauling routinely took 9,000 mg per day.

My point is that there is no exact value, and you have to establish for your own body an ongoing source of nutrients vital to proper function. Note that Vitamin C in your food is potentiated, or made much more effective by bioflavonoids, or separate chemicals in foods. Vitamin A is better sourced from food with its accompanying chemicals as well. It seems again that actual foods provide a better source of nutrients and less need for a label.

Processed food products also indicate milligrams of cholesterol. More recent studies, however, indicate that the cholesterol measured in your blood is much more closely tied to your carbohydrate intake and cholesterol and triglyceride production. Eating cholesterol for most people is not a big factor. In fact, in a simple lipid panel, more and more doctors are ignoring total cholesterol and looking at the ratio between the good cholesterol (HDL) and measured triglycerides as a measure of risk. Refer back to our discussion on lab testing for cardiovascular risk.

Even higher accuracy comes from the investigation of cholesterol particle size and number, along with other factors that indicate inflammation and lipoproteins known to cause damage. C-reactive protein, lipoprotein A, plaque indicators, thrombosis indicators, and other lab values tell a much more accurate story than total cholesterol. Most people can consume cholesterol and not even affect the blood values, since cholesterol is produced in the liver. What you really have to watch is your consumption of processed fats. Taking in good, natural fats take you several steps toward cardiovascular health.

Pay attention to the total amount of sugar that you consume and in what form you take it. It is very easy to consume a lot of high-fructose corn syrup or other processed sugars, or even mostly naturally occurring carbohydrates in high concentration. This is the case when you drink a lot of juices and smoothies. Don't just look at the foods that you consume. What about the sugar drinks, like sodas, or the salad dressings, ketchup, or the condiments. Account for all of it. Refer back to chapter 5 for more on how this affects you.

Finally, watch out for food additives. Chemicals are added to food as preservatives to enhance shelf life. You can even find pesticides in some snack foods. There are many chemicals added to food that will stimulate your senses and make you crave more, especially if the food doesn't have much nutritional value, and contains excitotoxins such as MSG.

Consuming whole vegetables and fruit in a limited quantity, has many health benefits. Even processing and juicing at home could pose problems. Be careful how much you sweeten beverages, since it is so easy to drink sugar down in high concentration. If you need more taste from your foods, it is probably a learned accommodation to stronger tastes, but you must be careful of damage to nerves and other structures. Get back to eating simple, unaltered food, and you'll find your taste buds again respond.

Chapter 11

The Supportive Cleanse

The Case for Cleansing

I eat healthy, exercise, and drink plenty of water. Is a cleanse really necessary?

The primary system of cleansing that I employ in the clinic is a supportive cleanse. We utilize a very basic hypoallergenic, low-inflammatory diet and supply nutrients beneficial to the detoxification process. Sometimes we include additional herbs for their anti-inflammatory or system-inducing properties. In either case, a cleanse must proceed long enough for the process to complete. I always like to arrange a seven-day cleanse up to optimally a twenty-eight-day cleanse. There are many variations of cleanse design, depending on the specific objective. However, we are not talking about a "medical cleanse," which is simply inducing a laxative effect so the colon is cleared for a medical procedure. Laxatives may be necessary to a cleanse, but the objective is to clear things from all body tissues. Along the same line of thinking, we do have to deal with constipation, because without regular bowel movements, the body will tend to reabsorb the materials left sitting in the large intestine or colon.

I would caution you to avoid short or severe cleanses (i.e., heavy doses of inducing herbs). It is difficult to properly cleanse the body safely in just two or three days. The shortest cleanse I will prescribe is seven to ten days. I prefer to have people cleansing for four weeks so that I am confident they have gone through all detoxification phases, including the excretion phase. The majority of the time I want people to do a supportive cleanse, I do not have them fast or even reduce calories to any great extent. I do specify what foods they are allowed to consume and also have them use a supplemental mix of nutrients to support the cleanse. It is also important that they avoid certain foods known to trigger an immune response. Generally, I will design a gluten-free, dairy-free, very clean diet, which is hypoallergenic.

If you choose to do a cleanse that requires a fast, very low-calorie intake, or the use of strong inducing herbs and laxatives, then pay attention to how you are tolerating it. A cleanse should never be overwhelming to you, even though some mild symptoms may occur. I can confidently state that every person that I have helped to design and implement a cleanse felt better after completing the detoxification process. I have seen cases of diabetes practically resolved with cleansing, dietary changes, and exercise.

Allergies, autoimmune disease, and even mental disorders respond very well to the cleansing process. If you let the body operate the way it is designed to, without the interference, problems just seem to resolve themselves. Sometimes all the prescribed medication just seems to make things worse, as the drugs themselves need to be detoxified. Through a cleanse you clear the medication load, as well as other toxic body burdens. When this is done, disease will be lessened or even nonexistent.

Under certain conditions, you will need to be cautious in proceeding with a cleanse. The cleanse may have to be modified in some way to control any negative effects, or perhaps not done at that time. If a woman desires to have a child, then she should do sufficient detoxification before conception. Once a woman knows she is carrying a developing fetus, cleansing is contraindicated, since this is not a good time to detoxify the mother's body. Cleansing will release toxins that will affect the development of the fetus and even deliver toxins directly to the child.

The same goes for mothers who are still nursing. Many toxic substances will be drawn from the mother's body and transferred to her milk, and then delivered to the breast-fed baby. In many ways, breastfeeding is beneficial for the developing child, but be aware that the mother will also excrete toxins from her body into the milk. Scientist now believe that even the placenta is not the barrier it was once thought to be, since toxins can cross the placenta barrier.

It is best to wait until a child is fully weaned before any mother attempts a detoxification regimen. Children themselves can also be especially sensitive to an induced detoxification. Caution must be taken to not overwhelm the young person's body. It has been shown that many children have accumulated many toxins at birth and during early life. The best strategy for children, though, is probably to allow their body to perform on its own by giving it the best nutrition possible. Many patients with chronic degenerative diseases will need to be careful with detoxification and cleansing systems, even though cleansing may be their best solution. A cleanse can still be done, but it must be modified so adverse reactions will be kept to a minimum.

In cases of cancer or tuberculosis, it is also important to be very careful with the type of cleanse done and the speed with which toxins are removed. In these cases where body systems are already compromised or not fully developed, the cleanse has to be more tailor made, if done at all. If designed carefully, cleansing is quite effective and helpful for your health and treatment of disease. However, we must keep in mind certain factors. Just how much exposure and toxic body burden does the person have to begin with? In the beginning, what is their state of health and how much can they tolerate? Any cleansing protocol can be modified to the situation. If the cleanse is started and the person exhibits overwhelming symptoms, or for other reasons it is too harsh or difficult, then it needs to be either modified or stopped completely.

The Clinical Supportive Cleanse: Cleanse Instructions

There are many levels of detoxification. The first is to eat a nontoxic diet composed of raw foods. A raw-foods diet contains lots of sprouted greens from seeds and grains, such as buckwheat, sunflower, alfalfa, clover, sprouted beans, and fresh vegetables. Raw foods maintain the highest concentration of vitamins, minerals, and important enzymes. Water should always be used during any type of detox program to help dilute and eliminate toxin accumulations. Supplementation is important to encourage healthy kidney and lymphatic system function, maintain healthy liver detoxification function, and promote efficient gastrointestinal elimination and blood purity. Supplementing with juniper berry, red clover flower, collinsonia root, psyllium husk, burdock root, barley grass, Spanish black radish root, fenugreek seed, fringe tree root, fennel seed, and milk thistle addresses the functioning of each detoxification system and supports the body's physiological functioning.

Colon cleansing is an important part of detoxification. Much toxicity comes out of the large intestine, and sluggish functioning of this organ can rapidly produce toxicity. To improve elimination through the skin, regular exercise is important to stimulate sweating, which aids in detoxification. Dry brushing the skin before bathing is suggested to cleanse the skin of old cells. Massage therapy, especially lymphatic and even deeper massage, is very useful in supporting a detox program; it stimulates elimination and body functions, and also promotes relaxation.

Step 1: Pre-Detoxification

If you drink caffeinated beverages, eat foods with high sugar content, or drink sodas (including diet), then you will need to reduce your consumption prior to starting the program. If you experience withdrawal from caffeine (i.e., headaches when you stop), we will have you wean off in decreasing amounts. During the cleanse period, you should not have sodas, coffee, candy, chocolates, etc., so begin limiting yourself prior to starting the cleanse. You can use naturally decaffeinated green teas and/or mineral water with unsweetened juice to make the transition easier. If you need to sweeten the tea, use stevia or xylitol (both found in most health-food stores).

Prepare your household by not having food you should avoid on hand. Begin throwing away all hydrogenated or partially hydrogenated oils and margarine, white sugar, artificial sweeteners, and refined white sugars and pastas. Stock your kitchen with the acceptable foods in the following charts so you will not be tempted to eat foods from the avoid list.

Water is another important component of the cleanse program. It is recommended that you consume at least half your body weight in ounces of water per day. Take your body weight in pounds and divide by two. That number is the minimum number of ounces of water you should drink every day. Example: Body weight = 120 pounds, 120/2 = 60; drink 60 ounces of water.

Step 2: Cleansing and Detoxification

The purpose of the cleanse is to give the body a period of rest. If you are not adding to your body burden and you give your body the right variety of nutrients, it will do what it is designed to do—eliminate substances from the body that are toxic and that interfere with function. We ask that you do a four-week cleanse process (see table below). We often prescribe a particular functional food (or cleanse product) with a good protein base, based upon health needs. This functional food is the primary dietary intake for one week of rest, otherwise it is supplemental. A good product can replace a meal or be consumed with other food. Please see below for a list of allowed foods.

General rules during cleanse:

- You may freely eat the foods listed, but you are asked to avoid some things as well.
- On days where cleanse drink servings are four or more per day, have a green vegetable (as much as you want) and the functional food only. Choose a different green vegetable each day.

- Eat a minimum of breakfast, lunch, and dinner. Try six smaller meals if you can schedule it. You can even simply graze throughout the whole day.
- A functional food serving is two scoops.
- The functional food can be used with a meal or take the place of a meal.
- We ask you to be careful of heating oils too high in cooking. Use a more stable oil like macadamia or coconut. It is best to cook with water, or bake or grill without oil. NO VEGETABLE OILS, CORN OIL, HYDROGENATED OIL, CRISCO, or PEANUT OIL!
- Soy products are acceptable in small amounts. A serving or two of soy milk or small amounts of miso or tempeh are preferable to processed soy products like tofu. Utilize other sources for protein as well.
- Consume organic or free-range products whenever possible.
- Drink plenty of clean, filtered water. Your goal is half your body weight in ounces per day.
- Eat two to three times as many vegetables as fruit (greater than 50 percent should be raw; if not raw, they should be lightly steamed or stir-fried over low heat).
- Avoid high glycemic index foods (foods that cause a fast rise in blood sugar), such as processed grains (even gluten free), corn, bananas, and white potatoes. Minimize or avoid tropical fruits.
- Salad dressing is permissible, but be sure to avoid those with corn syrup, fructose, dairy products, processed sugar, soy, or corn. Good choices are extra virgin olive oil, minced fresh garlic, lemon juice, sea salt, and black pepper.
- Avoid iodized salt. Celtic sea salt and Himalayan salt are acceptable, as long as the minerals are present.
- Avoid local lake fish. Purchase wild-caught fish. Do not fry. The amount should be the size and thickness of your palm. Occasionally you may have organic turkey or chicken, but ONLY

free range, antibiotic free, and hormone free. Baking or roasting is preferred to grilling or frying.

- Exercise is vital to health and, if enjoyed by the family, can lead to feelings of well-being and security. If you need to work up to this regimen or just weren't able to get it in on a certain day, take a minimum of a twenty- to thirty-minute walk.

Day 1 1 functional food Allowed food choices	**Day 2** 1 functional food Allowed food choices	**Day 3** 1 functional food Allowed food choices	**Day 4** 1 functional food Allowed food choices	**Day 5** 1 functional food Allowed food choices	**Day 6** 1 functional food Allowed food choices	**Day 7** 1 functional food Allowed food choices
Day 8 3 functional foods Allowed food choices	**Day 9** 3 functional foods 1 green vegetable (as much as desired)	**Day 10** 3 functional foods 1 green vegetable (as much as desired)	**Day 11** 3 functional foods 1 green vegetable (as much as desired)	**Day 12** 3 functional foods 1 green vegetable (as much as desired)	**Day 13** 3 functional foods 1 green vegetable (as much as desired)	**Day 14** 3 functional foods 1 green vegetable (as much as desired)
Day 15 1 functional food Allowed food choices	**Day 16** 1 functional food Allowed food choices	**Day 17** 1 functional food Allowed food choices	**Day18** 1 functional food Allowed food choices	**Day 19** 1 functional food Allowed food choices	**Day 20** 1 functional food Allowed food choices	**Day 21** 1 functional food Allowed food choices
Day 22 1 functional food Allowed food choices	**Day 23** 1 functional food Allowed food choices	**Day 24** 1 functional food Allowed food choices	**Day 25** 1 functional food Allowed food choices	**Day 26** 1 functional food Allowed food choices	**Day 27** 1 functional food Allowed food choices	**Day 28** 1 functional food Allowed food choices

FOOD GROUP	ALLOWED FOODS	DO NOT EAT
PROTEINS	Legumes except nuts (dried peas, lentils, etc.), cold water fish (salmon, halibut, mackerel, tuna, cod), chicken, turkey, lamb	Red meats, deli meats, frankfurters, sausage, canned meats, eggs and substitutes

DAIRY PRODUCTS	Use only unsweetened milk substitutes (rice milk, nut milks, soy milk, hemp milk, casein-free soy, rice or coconut products)	Milk, cottage cheese, yogurt, kefir, ice cream, cream, non-dairy creamers, casein, whey
STARCHES	Sweet potatoes, yams, arrowroot, rice, tapioca, buckwheat, millet, quinoa	All gluten-containing products including pasta, corn, and all corn-containing products
BREAD/ CEREAL	Minimally processed whole grain only: rice, quinoa, amaranth, buckwheat, teff, millet, soy, potato flour, tapioca, arrowroot	Wheat, oats, spelt, rye, barley
VEGETABLES	All colored, fibrous vegetables, preferably fresh or fresh frozen. Attempt to eat 5 servings or more and get all 5 colors	Creamed or canned anything made with prohibited ingredients
FRUITS	Unsweetened fresh or frozen. No juices and a ratio of 3 times as many vegetables	Fruit drinks, "ades," cocktails, citrus, strawberries, dried fruits
SOUP	Clear, vegetable-based broth; homemade vegetarian, chicken, or turkey soup; chili with chicken or turkey	Creamed or canned soups, or any soup or sauce containing gluten

BEVERAGES	Pure water, non-citrus herbal tea, mineral water. A small amount of unsweetened fruit juice or milk substitute can be mixed with cleanse drink if needed.	Milk, dairy based products, coffee, tea, cocoa, Postum, alcoholic beverages, soda, sweetened beverages, citrus drinks
FATS/OILS	Cold, expeller-pressed, unrefined, light-shielded canola oil, olive oil, grape seed oil, coconut oil. You can make your dressing with these	Margarine, shortening, butter, refined oils, salad dressings, spreads
NUTS/SEEDS	None	ALL nuts and seeds
SWEETENERS	Brown rice syrup, fruit sweeteners (agave), stevia, xylitol	Brown sugar, honey, molasses, maple syrup, fructose, sucrose, all artificial sweeteners
CONDIMENTS	Celtic/Himalayan salt (with minerals—NO iodized salt), salt-free herbs and seasonings, basil, cayenne pepper, caraway, chives, cinnamon, curry, dill, fry mustards, garlic, ginger, mace, marjoram, mint, nutmeg, parsley, poppyseed, savory	Salt, soy sauce, mayonnaise, ketchup

Recipe Ideas for Cleanse

Vegetable Soup

Sauté minced garlic and a chopped onion in minimum oil. Add 2 stalks of chopped celery and a diced green pepper. Add some vegetable broth (can purchase at Whole Foods), add some fresh herbs (cilantro, rosemary, etc.), and bring to a boil. Add vegetables of choice. Add delicate ones toward end (i.e., spinach, cabbage, etc.).

Baked Spaghetti Squash

Preheat oven to 375 degrees. With a long-tined fork, make deep pierces into the skin of the squash in several places and place in a baking dish. Bake for about 30 minutes, or until the skin is soft to touch. Cool for 10 minutes, cut in half lengthwise, and use a spoon to remove the seeds and strings from the center of the squash. Then use 2 forks to fluff up the flesh of the squash until you have spaghetti-like strands. Transfer strands to serving plates and top with herbs.

Ginger Lemonade

2 inches fresh ginger root

3 lemons

Stevia to taste

2 quarts of water

Wash and peel the ginger root. Grate it finely over a bowl. Squeeze the grated ginger mash with your fingers to extract the juice. Discard the dry mash. Bring water to a boil. Remove from heat and add ginger and juice of 3 lemons. Add stevia and stir well. Drink hot, or chill for iced ginger lemonade by adding ice cubes and a fresh slice of lemon.

Grilled Eggplant Slices

1 large eggplant (about 1¼ lbs)

2 cloves

3 tbsp extra virgin olive oil

¼ tsp sea salt

Freshly ground black pepper

Preheat gas grill on high. Slice eggplant 1/3–1/2 inch thick. In a small bowl, mix together the olive oil, garlic, salt, and pepper. Brush both sides of the eggplant slices with the mixture. Place eggplant on the preheated grill. If you wish to have nice grill lines, turn only once on each side. Grill eggplant slices 10–14 minutes.

Grilled Salmon Pepper Steaks

6 (6 oz) salmon steaks
¼ tsp sea salt
1/8 tsp pepper
2 tbsp fresh lemon juice
4 garlic cloves, minced
2 tbsp Dijon mustard
Olive oil
1 tbsp dark sesame oil
¼ tsp arrowroot

Sprinkle cracked pepper evenly over both sides of each salmon steak, and place steaks in a 13 x 9 inch baking dish. Combine next 5 ingredients in a small bowl; stir well. Pour mixture over steaks; cover and marinate in refrigerator 1 hour, turning steaks occasionally.

Prepare grill. Remove steaks from dish, reserving marinade. Place steaks on grill rack coated with olive oil, and grill 5 minutes on each side, basting frequently with half of reserved marinade. Combine remaining half of marinade and arrowroot in a small saucepan; bring to a boil and cook 1 minute or until thickened, stirring constantly with a wire whisk. Pour about 1 tbsp sauce over each steak. Makes 6 servings.

Blackened Ahi Tuna

Make sure you buy the freshest possible sashimi-grade tuna, and serve it rare or medium rare for the best flavor. Sear the fish in a cast-iron skillet, so that it is cooked on the outside but still pink on the inside.

4 (7 oz) center cut ahi tuna filets
½ tsp fresh ginger root

½ tsp each sea salt and garlic powder

½ tsp fresh garlic, paprika, onion powder

½ tsp each black pepper and white pepper

1 dash fresh lime juice

1/8 tsp each cayenne pepper, thyme, and oregano

3/4 c olive oil

2 tbsp wasabi

3 fl oz water

Preheat cast iron skillet. Rub fillets with Cajun blackening spice. Sear both sides (no butter or oil needed) until rare or medium rare. Cut filet into 2 triangular pieces; overlap.

(To make Cajun blackening spice: combine salt, garlic powder, paprika, onion powder, black pepper, white pepper, cayenne pepper, thyme, and oregano; mix well.)

Combine wasabi with water and put in blender. Add grated ginger, garlic, white wine vinegar, and lime juice into the blender and drizzle in oil while on high speed. Adjust seasoning with salt and pepper.

Fantastic Halibut

Start to marinate the fish at least 2 hours before you plan to serve it.

3 cloves garlic, minced

1 tsp pepper

1 tbsp olive oil

¼ c fresh lime juice

1¼ c fresh basil, chopped

1½ lbs halibut fillets or steaks

1 tbsp sea salt

Combine all ingredients, except for fish, in a shallow dish large enough to hold the halibut. Place fish in the dish and marinate for at least 2 hours, turning once or twice. Remove fish from marinade and broil or grill for about 5 minutes on each side (10 minutes total per inch of thickness). Transfer fish to a serving dish. Heat remaining marinade in a saucepan; pour over fish. Serve while hot.

Roasted Chicken with Herbs

Easy and fast. Serve with vegetables or salad.

2 lbs broiler chicken, uncooked

1 tbsp fresh sage (or dried)

3 cloves garlic, minced

½ tsp sea salt

1 tbsp fresh thyme leaves (or dried)

½ tsp freshly ground pepper

½ tbsp fresh rosemary leaves (or dried)

Preheat oven to 350 degrees. If using fresh herbs, remove leaves with stems and chop. Combine minced garlic, thyme, rosemary, sage, salt, and pepper in a small bowl. Wash chicken under cold water, trim excess fat, and pat dry with paper towels. Starting at the neck cavity, loosen skin from breast and drumsticks by inserting fingers, gently pushing between skin and meat. Rub herb mixture under loosened skin. Place chicken in a shallow roasting pan coated with olive oil. Bake for about 1 hour. Cover loosely with cloth and let stand for 5–10 minutes before carving. Discard skin, carve, and serve.

Part Four

Stress and the Healthy Mind

Chapter 12

The Case for Functional Mind

To have a healthy mind requires that you have a healthy body. One cannot work independently of the other. Millions of dollars are spent on drugs for the mind and "head doctors," i.e., specialists like psychiatrists, each year. Another group of doctors, "body doctors," specialize in treatments for the body. To understand the whole picture, we have to get the specialists together and realize that mind and body are not separate. Medication in conjunction with good psychotherapy can be very helpful tools. People are better able to cope and handle stress when they feel better both mentally and physically. I believe that both mental and physical problems can be resolved with the right strategy and approach. Just like we have discussed for the body, we want to strive for the freedom and independence of being healthy in mind as well.

I wonder sometimes about people who seem to assume that the mind and body are not really connected. To understand how the body works is to understand how all these biological systems work together.

If you're going to treat the mind, then you absolutely must treat the body, and vice versa. However, the continuing theme of this book is that the treatment really is something you do best for yourself. If you experience mental/emotional control issues, I encourage you to look into rehabilitation and recovery for your body wellness and not get too involved in treatment of mental dysfunction by itself. Look for patterns that relate to whole body function.

Many pharmaceutical medications are designed to control mental function and, for the most part, keep a person's behaviors acceptable within society. This can also be a real advantage for people themselves to be able to cope with the stress and anxiety often occurring in our lives. Unfortunately there are cases where it has become, and is actually referred to as, a form of chemical incarceration. In times past, people were ostracized, asked to leave the community, sent away on the "ship of fools," or banished and even ex-communicated. Some were actually put to death for thinking or being different. Later in time, perhaps a person who did not conform, or fit in, would be placed in an institution such as an asylum. However, now we use modern chemistry to exert control. We can give someone a pill so that they will behave properly. Perhaps more alarming than this is the fact that so many people are prescribed these drugs to cope with their day-to-day lives. At times this might be appropriate, but it also creates an unwanted dependence on and belief in medication.

Yes, people on pharmaceutical drugs are better able to control themselves and may be able to function more appropriately in society. This is instead of locking them up in asylums and institutions where they were often used for experiments. Maybe it is better for society, but is it truly better for the patients? Are they still no more than an experiment? In fact, many more people are administered these drugs as a convenience. For example, your general practitioner might prescribe for you a certain drug because you sound a little depressed. Sometimes emotions are appropriate and fit your current situation. It might be better to simply experience the moods and emotions in order to move past them. Regardless, if you get your body functioning better, your brain function improves at the same time. You will never experience a healthy mind with an unhealthy body.

Many professionals have adopted the belief that people need, and cannot live without, brain-altering chemicals throughout their life. This belief assumes that your only choice is to introduce foreign chemicals to control your brain and emotions. There are many ways to produce healthy mental functioning and healthy chemistry. What people really need is comprehensive mind and body health, not the prospect of needing drugs for their lifetime. Many psychiatrists will actually tell people that they have no other choice but to take the medications prescribed and continue to see the practitioner without end. It is an absolute fact that drugs can be useful, especially in the short term; however, they are not necessary to human life. They are simply tools that can be helpful at certain times. By far the best answer to good mental health is proper function of your body physiology.

Your digestive tract actually produces more neurotransmitters in quantity than your brain does. Health is the result of the whole human body functioning optimally. In order to have health in the brain, it is imperative that you have a healthy body, especially a healthy gut. We can manipulate our brain chemistry, emotions, focus, and moods with drugs, or we can improve our digestive function and have a similar impact without the drug. So much begins in the gastrointestinal tract. This is a point of major interaction with the environment. It is where substances are introduced into the body, and where the body must sample and discriminate as to what to let in and what to keep out. If too many toxins are allowed in, this will also interfere with brain chemistry and the mind. If there are too few nutrients absorbed, this will affect the brain and its function as well. If the body gets the wrong messages, substances are produced in the digestive tract that are destined to affect mental function.

The body will do what it is designed to do. Optimize nutrition, and you enhance mental function. I don't mean consuming a few vegetables here and there; I mean that you have to take in an optimal amount of nutrients so that your body has the right materials and cofactors to work with. If you spend your day eating only empty calories, lacking these nutrients, then the body and the mind will be unable to function. You can improve function by taking in natural healthy fats, or destroy it by consuming altered, unnatural fats. If you lack the right balance of amino acids, you can severely affect moods and mental function. Many studies on Alzheimer's indicate that the incidence of Alzheimer's is much higher among people who consume high-calorie, low-nutrient diets. People who consumed more vegetables, good protein, and fats, and were closer to the Mediterranean diet, experienced a much lower incidence of Alzheimer's and other dementias.

If hormones are produced and available at the right physiological levels, the receptors are functioning, and the hormones are broken down properly, then you create proper mental and physical function. When hormones fluctuate abnormally, symptoms will occur. Certain hormones actually act to protect your neurological systems, most notably the brain itself, and affect repair in case of damage. Other hormones acting as messengers keep the body and the mind running smoothly. This means the mind is dependent on balance in the body. We all benefit when we have the right physiological levels of bio-identical hormones. Estrogen and progesterone are known to be neuro-protective molecules and are also proven to be cardio-protective, keeping your heart safe. Testosterone helps in the renewal of nerve cells and other body cells and tissues. If your hormones become deficient and the neural network is not protected, then damage will take place.

If inflammation is not kept under control in the body, then there will be damage to the brain as well. The brain is often the most susceptible tissue, and of course this has a large impact on mental functions such as memory and cognition. When you allow unrestricted inflammation to occur, you also allow damage and dysfunction to occur throughout the body. In fact, all mental disorders demonstrate evidence of brain inflammation. If you're not controlling inflammation, you are facilitating the collateral damage that will occur as well in the brain. Most, if not all, brain disorders are tied to this uncontrolled inflammation. Yet a large number of people in our society are found to have ongoing evidence of inflammation—which is not even addressed during their treatment for mental and emotional disorders.

Autoimmune disease is being diagnosed at an all-time high. Autoimmunity seems to be a result of the same mechanism, exhibiting differently depending on the tissues that are inflamed. If inflammation occurs in the brain, then you will experience brain disorders. Many neurological and mental/emotional disorders are autoimmune disease in the brain. On many occasions, when treating autoimmune disorders such as rheumatoid arthritis, Hashimoto's thyroiditis, Sjogren's and others, there is also a great improvement in depression, focus, concentration, and other symptoms that were thought to be only problems of the mind.

Many regard your digestive tract as still being outside of the body. It contains a large portion of your immune system. It is the place where food is broken down into nutrients and then absorbed, but it also serves as a final border to the bloodstream. As your body cells sample your food, they discover things that could hurt you if they got into the bloodstream. When a foreigner is identified, access to the blood is hopefully blocked, and the body mounts an immune response to keep you safe. If your digestive system becomes a source of inflammation, this will lead again to dysfunction of your brain as the foreign substances travel to the brain. If the gut isn't functioning well, neither is your body, and neither is your mind. Mental health requires brain health. Control of emotions will only be possible when the brain can function normally with the balance of molecular chemistry.

Proper detoxification must be taking place to allow the transformation and elimination of substances and molecules dangerous to the body—dangerous because in many cases they interfere with normal function itself. Foreign substances create an inflammatory response and, in some cases, directly damage tissue or impair function. For example, we've mentioned that if mercury is present, it has the ability to destroy the myelin sheath covering the nerves. Multiple sclerosis is known to be an autoimmune disorder, and in a number of cases mercury was implicated as a cause of

MS symptoms. As we learned in the chapters on detoxification, very often the lack of concentration or focus, or "foggy thinking," is a product of the total body burden of toxins in the body. We have had many cases of mental improvement right after someone finishes a cleansing protocol for the body.

The most common physical symptom people report when starting at our clinic is being fatigued. Fatigue comes down to an interference to the system of energy production called the Krebs cycle and electron transport chain. When you are fatigued, the brain is out of energy. We all know what it feels like to experience fatigue. Of course, it is very difficult to do anything requiring physical exertion because of this. Perhaps more importantly, though, without energy your brain is just not able to function in normal fashion. This will lead to problems with concentration and emotions. Remember a time when you skipped some meals and found yourself to be less productive? Perhaps you observed that emotional balance and moods were also affected. With low energy, you might be depressed, angry, and even somewhat schizophrenic. But you did not have a clinical disease pathology; your mind was demanding energy to function. Give your brain the energy it needs, and you will find that it functions very well.

Stress creates mental problems that we all have experienced. If you allow the stress response to run unchecked, you actually end up doing physical damage to your own neural network. If you feel stressed all the time, then you are living in a situation called sympathetic dominance. Unfortunately, many people live out their entire lives this way. Eventually they become overwhelmed or burned out, and they begin developing many chronic diseases because their body is actually worn out. We all have a real need for down time and recovery. For many people, an effective amount of sleep has become difficult to obtain—sometimes as a result of scheduling, and other times as a result of poor health. In either case, if you don't sleep, and you don't give your body adequate recovery time, you will also become mentally unfit.

When we use up all of our resources and don't allow proper recovery of our mind or our body, we will not function properly. Sympathetic dominance is the situation where your mind just will not turn off. You remain in your sympathetic state, or fight or flight state, constantly. Neither your mind nor your body is able to cope with ongoing stress. The hormones and neurotransmitters that form your stress response are necessary when you need to take action. However, these same molecules produced in your body will turn on you and create damage if not utilized properly. We all need to be aware to not be on all the time, or we are driving ourselves to exhaustion. It is good to learn how to utilize your parasympathetic nervous system for the rest and recovery of your brain and body.

This is a very important concept to wrap your head around. Animals, when studied in their natural environment, are often put in situations where they are dealing with stress. An animal running for its life to escape a predator, or a predator trying to obtain necessary food, enters a state of stress. We are talking about life or death situations. The difference between the animals and human beings is that the animal takes physical action (fight or flight—either running for its life to get away or chasing prey for the food to stay alive. The physical response of fight or flight is actually the answer to avoiding the negative consequences of stress. Animals, when studied in natural conditions, showed no adverse affects from the stress itself, as long as they take physical action and then have a bit of down time.

Human beings, on the other hand, tend to be relatively inactive, even though they stimulate the same physiological response. We understand some stimulus(stress), and we live in the same condition of fight or flight. It is a very similar response to life stresses. Without the actual physical response to fight or flight, the stress response begins to affect our health. Physical damage occurs to the human being who sits and frets. The best answer to avoid negative effects from stress is physical activity. Your stress response is preparing you to take action. If you don't respond appropriately, you will end up with a physical and mental illness. Almost anyone might be found to have a mental disorder under the right conditions. (We'll talk more about this dynamic in the next chapter.)

Without physical activity, stress hormones and other chemicals are still released, and if not put to use for activity (response), they begin to cause dysregulation of glucose metabolism and damage your neural network. There is evidence of these effects of stress damaging the brain and causing Alzheimer's disease. Other neural damage may relate to a number of mental and physical disorders. Stress is a component of life, and you can use it in many positive ways. If you don't learn to use it correctly, stress will do damage to your mind and body. When you are stressed, I heartily recommend that you get up and move.

It really comes back to a lifestyle that fits you and maintains, or even improves, your health. It is really better for you to learn what real food is and consume primarily that. You know better than any practitioner when something is working and when it is not. Experiment and understand the types of food you are better suited for, even to the point of understanding your own ancestors and what they ate. They adapted to the best diet for their own situation, and this absolutely has an effect on you. You will likely have to consume enough vegetables to benefit from their nutrients. You will have to consume sufficient protein of high-enough quality. Some fruit can be beneficial as well. Remember to apply the principles of physical activity when you're stressed. Your exercise or activity routine will have to be consistent, challenging, and of sufficient variety to produce results.

Understand that the primary drug that you will ever take in is actually the food you will consume throughout your lifetime. Good nutrition delivers good communication to the body. When you communicate the right messages to the body, you end up with better results. There is a real and present need for nutrients, but you also need your connection to the outside world through xenohormeosis, which we previously discussed. However, xenohormetic effects can be negative too. A very small amount of the wrong substance from the environment might really impair brain function. In my opinion, it is much better to work on clearing out interference than it is to add more interfering chemicals (even medications).

Insomnia is perpetuated by our modern diet and our modern schedules, which promote living the sympathetic-dominant lifestyle with chaotic schedules and no balance in hormones. Sympathetic dominance occurs when you don't spend some time with the parasympathetic. Remember that the autonomic nervous system is that part of your nervous system that is not voluntary, and it consists of a sympathetic system and a parasympathetic system. The voluntary system is under your control, an example being the contraction of a muscle to move your arm. The sympathetic branch is your fight or flight system, which responds to any stress. If you count yourself as a "type A" personality, or you know that you cannot turn off your brain even for sleep, then you are sympathetic dominant.

The parasympathetic system allows you rest and recovery. Digestion and elimination, sleep, tissue repair, sex, and reproduction are examples of parasympathetic function. If you are sympathetic dominant, you don't enjoy those functions or do them well. There are functions that bridge these two systems, and two notable ones are breathing and exercise. The act of breathing can be accomplished voluntarily, as when you take an intentional deep breath. What about when you sleep, or are not paying attention—will you die if you forget to breathe for very long? That is when the autonomic nervous system takes over for you and keeps you breathing.

A great breathing exercise for kids, and adults as well, is to envision a candle burning in front of you. Inhale through your nose to a slow count of four, so that you draw the flame and the smoke in your direction. Hold your breath for another slow count of four, and then breathe out through your mouth strong enough to move the flame and smoke away from you, but not blow the candle out, in a final count of four. You can repeat this several times to facilitate a calming down from anxiety.

Breathing can be a very effective tool for the control of panic disorders (PTSD), anxiety, and control of depression. When you are in the sympathetic state, it is easy to lose control of emotions; with a simple breathing exercise you can bring your physiology into the parasympathetic, where you can relax and regain control. Another very effective way to get from sympathetic to the parasympathetic is exercise. When you exercise, you are utilizing your sympathetic system; however, as soon as you stop exercising, you have a guaranteed reflex into the parasympathetic so you can recover. If your sympathetic dominance comes only from stressful mental functions, you do not have an easy route to the parasympathetic until you reach complete exhaustion. So wellness is about creating balance, even in how you use the nervous system of the body.

So if you're even too stressed to get quality sleep, then you will always be running behind. When you don't sleep well, the primary thing to consider is sleep hygiene: your sleeping schedule, your sleeping space, and your inability to access the parasympathetic system. If we don't schedule a time for sleep, actually making a date with the bed on a regular schedule, then your body and your mind don't know when to be alert or when to recover. When you stay awake and when you make schedule changes, your body tries to accommodate you by producing cortisol to keep you alert. Then when you want to sleep, you will need to be able to produce melatonin.

We all need on the average about seven-and-a-half hours of sleep. We generally need three cycles into deep, or REM, sleep to be ready for the next waking period. If the balance and scheduling of cortisol and melatonin is not reliable, then neither is your state of health. When you don't get good quality sleep on a regular basis, you will lose mental function and health. It behooves you to support your daily or diurnal cycle. The best way to do this is to keep a consistent schedule and use your parasympathetic system. Your brain needs rest and recovery just like your body does. Without good sleeping habits and without enough physical activity, you just can't get into a good recovery state.

Hormonal imbalance not only interrupts sleep but many other processes as well. Most hormonal symptoms stem from the fluctuation hormones, rather than just absolute higher or lower levels. In every case, when hormones are not in balance with each other, the body cannot be healthy since the proper messages are not delivered. Thyroid, insulin, estrogen, testosterone, glucagon, and progesterone are just a few of the important hormones that need to be in balance with each other. If you cause changes in one, then you have had an impact on all of them.

Inflammation must be controlled. If your brain or any part of your body are under an immune response, they are literally on fire. If you don't get this under control, the effects can become extreme and often leads to autoimmunity. Autoimmunity is now rampant in our culture, when it used to be almost unheard of. Rheumatoid arthritis, lupus, Sjogren's, Hashimoto's, and the list goes on. Interestingly, these diseases are related in their mechanism. The immune system has basically gone rogue. No longer able to discern your tissues from foreign invaders, your immune system begins to attack your own tissues. The process exhibits in different ways depending on the tissue affected or attacked. Autoimmune disease is created from this dysfunction. It is very closely related to diet, physical activity, and allergic response.

Heart disease is increasingly more common. Arterial damage, circulation problems, and high blood pressure are all very much affected by your lifestyle. Here we go again: your eating habits and your lack of physical activity, bringing you into chronic disease. Heart disease and stroke are causative factors of mental dysfunction as well as sometimes permanent damage. Circulation is extremely important for the brain to function. Your focus, concentration, and even your memories require energy production, circulation, and control of inflammation.

Diabetes, especially adult onset or type II, is considered a lifestyle disease. The more scientists learn about diabetes, the closer we are to the conclusion that the mechanism of creation comes from lifestyle, especially the frequent fluctuations in blood sugar. Sugar causes dysfunction and damage in the brain itself.

Cancer, once thought to come out of nowhere, is now understood as a mechanism. In fact, the "war" on cancer has not been won after all this time and probably never will. As we mentioned before, modern scientists are beginning to understand that the solution to cancer is to not allow an environment to be created where cancer can flourish. Cancer doctors can have success if they debulk, or remove enough of, the cancer for the body to finish the job.

Many of the healthiest people I know are cancer survivors. Whether or not they had to undergo cancer treatment, their real success came from a change in lifestyle. Upon hearing that they had cancer, they got busy with improving their health: changing eating habits drastically, including daily physical exercise, and paying better attention to environmental exposures. These changes did not happen overnight, but they were most productive in cancer remission or shortening the duration of treatment.

The human body is a collection of biological systems completely interrelated and absolutely dependent on one another. Any single system can be responsible for the diseases currently described in conventional medical management. In functional medicine, which I want you to be a student of, we look for patterns and clues that tell us how well the systems are working together and also where the actual source of the problem may be found. For example, in mental disease, I often find that when I have amino-acid levels tested, there is almost always a significant imbalance. When I work with the digestive system, helping it to heal and improve its function, and at the same time give the patient amino acids found lacking in their free form, I can restore amino-acid balance in the body. In many if not all cases, mental functioning improved, and sometimes mental and emotional problems would resolve altogether.

After dividing the systems of the body up to study them and create specialties, scientists now have to go back and understand what happens when the systems are operating in the body together at the same time. Thus we have new areas of study. One of the newest on the forefront is the science of the neuroendocrineimmune system. Your nervous system, your hormones, and your immune system actually interact with each other in many ways. Information is gathered and responses are driven all within a common feedback loop. If you figuratively say that you can't stomach something, you are still being literal. Because when you think about something distasteful, there is an actual gut and nervous-system response.

We will talk more about stress in the next chapter. I do want to make another mention of it here, though. When you are under more stress than the body can handle, that is when you begin to exhibit symptoms. This holds true for both physical and mental symptoms. So if you commonly experience stress, and that stress creates a symptom like a headache, then you are very likely living too close to your threshold volume of stress. We will talk further about finding ways to utilize stress for adaptation and not let stress do harm to you. When you understand stress, you can use it advantageously. However, you also have to learn how to mediate stress effects, or it will also lead to dysfunction.

There are a few things that are not productive for stress relief. One is to eat in order to alleviate stress. Food, except for alleviating hunger and lack of nutrients, will not positively impact stress. There are better methods for stress relief, especially exercise. Emotional eating is eating while you have the poorest judgment. The things that you will tend to consume probably have no health benefits at all. Who grabs broccoli when they are stressed? Most likely it is a pint of ice cream, or a can of frosting, or perhaps popcorn or some other snack. These choices may serve to increase serotonin a bit, but the long-term effects will be negative. I don't know anyone who can make good choices or eat good foods when they are stressed. We all tend to gravitate to the sugar and the junk.

That lack of control leads to a situation that eventually becomes diabetes. Cholesterol rises, triglycerides rise, insulin levels are higher since more is required, and hormones are pushed out of balance. You begin to accumulate weight. But more importantly, you create mental and emotional dysregulation. Start by using the glycemic index to judge every food that you eat. Start exercising, since exercise alone can stimulate the transport of sugar as well as increase insulin sensitivity. What this leads to is better control with less mental dysfunction and disease.

Have you ever been to the zoo? Do you remember the sign that read "don't feed the animals"? Essentially what it really said was "don't feed the animals what you are eating, because it will hurt them, or even kill them." If your food choices are unfit for animals to eat, maybe you should consider eating food that won't hurt you either.

Every one of these chronic diseases that we are discussing have a direct effect on your mental and emotional health. Many behaviors that are described as mental disorders seem to virtually disappear when you improve these chronic diseases. When you get the body functioning better, disorders of the mind to seem to just fade away. In fact, most mental disorders have no actual laboratory evidence or pathological existence. They are simply behaviors observed and classified by a practitioner. Concentrate on physical health, and you likely will not have to worry about mental and emotional disorders.

Let me finish this chapter by again stating that if you don't feel good physically, you are also off-balance mentally. Many people diagnosed with mental disorders simply don't feel good. Think about your own experience with your focus, concentration, and your mental state. When people are physically sick, we would very likely diagnose him with some mental disorder, unless we knew them and their psyche at a point when they were well. I have seen remarkable changes in people as they transition from the physical problems. Even on a weight-loss program, there is not just a change in physical appearance. Most of these people exhibit drastic changes in their mental outlook. Many were very depressed, with a number coming in taking several medications, but by the end of the program and having lost some weight, they no longer needed the medication. So did they have a mental disease, or not?

Chapter 13

Stress for Success

Stress might be simply defined as anything that places us "off balance." The balance that I am referring to is both physical as well as mental. When the body perceives the force of stress, that stress is analyzed, readings are taken within and throughout the body, and the best response available at the time is produced. This is unless we focus mentally and change or stop the response. I could be speaking about simply losing your balance if someone pushes you, and you fall. Even in that example, proprioception, biochemical analysis, shifts in physiology, and other measures led to judgments, reaction, and a response. However, there are few limits to stresses and the responses to them.

We can physically and mentally adapt to a stressor. The alternative is to remain out of balance, degenerate, or breakdown. The better that we understand stress, our adaptation to it, and how the body will be reset or change, the more we can actually learn to benefit from stress itself. Generally, we think of stress as something that affects us mentally.

However, the original definition of stress was all about measuring physical forces acting upon physical inanimate objects—for example, the stress that a bridge might withstand as it holds up objects that are transported across it. Dr. Hans Selye took the original description of stress and applied it to living things.

Dr. Selye described stress as hunger, thirst, pain, work, and even nutritional deficiency. Stress produces changes in each animal's biochemistry, and mentally perceived stresses seemed to create the same physiological results as a physical stress. In essence, stress is any force acting upon an inanimate object, or both the perceived and real forces upon a living being. This "force" has the effect of throwing us out of balance. In the human being, stress is any force generated physically or mentally that creates an imbalance to which the body must respond. The human body can respond to stress by resisting and correcting the imbalance, or it may succumb to it. When the body is exposed to stress, this will lead to the production of some response.

For example, starvation and extreme diets place a significant stress on the body, since the body suddenly realizes that nutrients and calories are in short supply. In fact, people are obsessed with dieting in our society, and most people's concept of a diet is to simply eat less to the point of creating starvation. People are so concerned about their appearance and will go to great lengths in an attempt to control how they look. Of course, most people do not want to put the time and effort into doing this in a safe and effective manner. They will look in the mirror, or someone may mention that they are starting to gain weight. Their response is a decision to go on a crash diet for quick results.

In fact, since they desire immediate gratification, it is a common decision to begin a period of fasting and starvation. We call it skipping meals, but any period of "famine" has the same effect as starvation. The body reads the stress that there is suddenly less nutrients and calories available, or perhaps no intake at all. At this point, the body begins to make adjustments and change set points as its response to this new situation of famine. These adjustments will very soon become adaptations, actual changes in body structure and physiology that you will have to live with.

Let's just say that you are skipping meals hoping to lose weight quickly, and you are excited when the scale goes down. But what weight did you really lose? It is very likely that, if you reduce your caloric intake drastically, you will end up burning muscle, bone tissue, and organ tissue for fuel, but not the fat you wanted to lose. This is because your body believes that there is a famine, and it must prepare a response. Your body does not know that there is a supermarket right around the corner. What the body perceives as a fact is that no food could mean starvation and death. The body begins to adjust and adapt as it formulates a response to the stress. This response will include increasing cortisol production, changing body organ function, altering hormone levels, and doing anything and everything to survive in a period of famine.

In a starvation situation, the body attempts to do more with less. A logical response, then, is to slow down the metabolic rate. One direct effect is on the thyroid gland, since thyroid hormones are directly responsible for the basal metabolic rate and temperature regulation, as well as orchestrating other systems. Your body actually resets thyroid function so that you will not need as many calories. This means that when you begin to eat again, you will be less able to maintain your weight. The thyroid was adjusted to adjust your metabolism and your ability to generate energy and heat. Now you have created a situation that is hypothyroidism. Don't be deceived because the scale indicated a lower number of pounds. The healthy objective is to change body composition, maintaining muscle, bone, and your internal organs, and preferentially metabolizing your fat stores. We want to be "lean and mean," not "skinny and fatigued."

With less weight, you might not look quite the way that you intended to, but at least you're in smaller-sized clothes. What actually happened is that you lost muscle and retained fat, and now you are off the diet as an unwell person. You begin to gain weight back faster than you lost it. You are now proportionally fatter than you were before. Your body doesn't work as well with more fat and less lean tissue. Worse than that, your thyroid is now reset, and your metabolism is actually slower. At least your body demonstrated that it can adapt to the stress.

A much better plan is referred to as caloric restriction. Remember, this is not starvation. Caloric restriction is defined as less calorie intake along with more nutrients. What we want to avoid is placing the body into a situation where the nutrients are deficient. In deficiency, the body has to break itself down to find nutrients (become catabolic) in order to function. Some very good studies demonstrate that a 20- to 30-percent decrease in caloric intake, with proper levels of nutrient intake, has the ability to improve health and even lengthen lifespan.

Another example of how you might adapt and reset something that was working well before as a result of stress is your daily cycle. The diurnal cycle of the body, or its circadian rhythm, is primarily determined by two important hormones. Cortisol is an adrenal hormone that is produced in the morning and is responsible for awaking you from sleep. The cortisol level is normally highest first thing in the morning, and then slowly falls off to a low point, just before it is time for you to sleep. At that point, melatonin is produced and follows a similar pattern through the night, having as many as three peak amounts to facilitate the three normal cycles into REM sleep. Many people detrimentally affect this cycle when they don't keep a consistent schedule. Our goal in health is more than increasing the lifespan; what we want is health span, or quality of life, while we are here.

Let's say that you keep a normally consistent schedule, which actually promotes healthy function. Something out of the ordinary comes up, perhaps a book to read, a movie you'd like to finish, a project due for school or work, or just more to do than you had time to do during the day. Now you make a conscious decision to stay up past your bedtime. We will say that normally your bedtime is 10:30 p.m., but you're struggling to stay up, and now it is after midnight. Out of the blue, you find that you've gotten a "second wind." How fortunate; now you are wide awake, and you can finish everything that you wanted to do. What just happened? Well, your body perceived that you wanted to stay up, and it was happy to give you a dose of cortisol. This was a proper physiological response to the stress, but it happened in the middle of the night.

That one dose of cortisol may be enough, or this may have to go on for a few nights. In either case, it is not too long before this stress response will remain, and now you can rely on that middle-of-the-night cortisol to wake you up at night when you want to sleep. I want you to sleep right for your health, and you want to sleep as you did before, but your body has a new schedule in place. What are you going to do now? Will you take a sleeping pill or see a doctor? The best answer is to restore the original schedule and learn about sleep hygiene. You may have to make a date with your bed and stay there in the dark for a few nights. Create a good sleeping space, with no distractions, and reestablish a better hormone-production pattern. This can be done, and you are resetting your own clock. Unfortunately, sleep medication will only knock you out; it will not reset your hormones. All medication can do is induce coma; it cannot create a natural sleep that lets the body restore itself. Only you can do that.

Stress is absolutely unavoidable, and it will be present from the day that you are born to the day that you die. In fact, stress continues even beyond the grave. Even as you die and decompose there is stress on your body, as the molecules that made it up decompose. Everyone must deal with stress, and everyone is affected by stress. The best strategy will be to learn how to use it to create positive and healthy adaptations. Stress in itself is actually neither good nor bad. The amount of stress experienced, and the physiological reaction to the stress, tells the tale. We all have a choice to either use it in a positive way, or to let it destroy us.

It is quite possible to learn control over the amount of stress affecting us, and how we experience it. The eventual response to stress will be one of either adaptation, or maladaptation. Adaptation is seen as the positive response to stress. People are stressed in their relationships, in financial situations, when they don't have enough time, when driving in traffic, even when they skip meals or don't get enough fluids. Maladaptive responses are the negative results which occur when we are under too much stress and are unprepared for it. The ultimate goal is to learn about stress, and then to use it for benefit. This is a major secret to success is in life.

"May the Force Be with You"

If stress is only recognized as an emotional force, then we will misinterpret the physical forces acting upon our physical bodies. Exercise and activity are stress, nutrition is a stress, and natural forces like sun, wind, and rain are stressors. Stress will act upon you whether you want it to or not. However, many stresses are, in fact, something that you can control. The first step for all of us is to understand which stresses we have control over, and those that we do not. We must all be careful not to be led astray, like Don Quixote chasing windmills. It takes an awareness of what things we can really exert our power upon, so that we don't waste talent, time, and energy on things we cannot change. There are still many effective battles to be waged upon the things we can do something about. Even better, when we understand the effect of the stress, we can actually utilize it to make us better (adapt).

The realization that stress has a much broader scope than simply mental anxiety is a source for hope. A better understanding of stress creates a tool for change for the better. Hans Selye, who coined the term "stress," was describing the total stress experienced in a lifetime, from all sources. Stress comes in many forms and is ultimately anything that throws the body off balance, or anything that produces a response. In someone with a healthy, well-functioning body, that response is small yet effective, and almost unnoticed. In many cases, through adaptation, your response lessens each time you experience similar stress. This is viewed as a positive force for change. In others, whose bodies are not functioning as well, the stress response is often greater, produces physical damage, and possibly creates maladaptation or further dysfunction.

For example, take someone training for a running race, perhaps a marathon. If that person trains and conditions their body through the planned application of stress, they will be ready. Readiness means a body rebuilt for speed, stability, resistance to injury, and of course endurance. If they applied the force of stress correctly, they will complete the race, enjoy the race, and perhaps even produce a personal best time of performance. However, without this application of force of training, another person will not make physical changes or adaptations in their body that will allow them to participate in the race in the same way. Likely the second person will not even finish the race. It is not about practice; it is about applying the right forces that change physical structures and function.

Negative stress stems from poor nutrition, poor hydration, and in essence a poorly planned and executed lifestyle. Resilience to stress stems from a lifestyle that is congruent with a healthy body. If your body does not get all the nutrients that it requires, then stress is created as your body tries to respond with these limitations in place. Without the requisite nutrients to proceed and function in a healthy manner, the body must make critical decisions in its attempt to, at minimum, sustain your life. However, the body is limited in the resources necessary to produce vitality or optimum health. When we don't provide all the nutrients that our body requires, your physiology will attempt to function at the best level possible, but now with limitations. Placing restrictions on how well your body can function is the way that we erode health, create symptoms, and eventually develop disease. Our bodies will adapt, in an attempt to function best under the present situation. Poor adaptation actually limits our ability to function normally and to be healthy.

Exercise and physical activity present stresses for the body to deal with and then adapt to. Exercise, planned out and executed properly, is an extremely positive force for change. It stimulates our bodies to adapt and be able to accommodate more stress than before. Physical activity does actually lead to metamorphosis of the body. Exercise will make us bigger, faster, stronger, smarter, and more graceful and coordinated. Perhaps the most important effect that we gain from exercise is the increased production of energy. When we exercise, we are demanding more energy. If we exercise to a degree that is challenging to our bodies, then the body will adapt by finding a way to provide that energy. This is the proper use of the "force."

We've defined organ reserve as the resilience that the human body demonstrates when it is healthy. Many problems blamed on aging are only a loss of organ reserve. You can increase organ reserve by applying stress correctly, and cause the body to adapt so that succeeding stresses require less effort in response. There is stress placed on muscles, bones, and your internal organs when you ask them to perform in any way. The ability of these body tissues to respond is a measure of your organ reserve. When the body works better, it can handle more stress, since it is more capable and efficient. The response is now adequate and timely. When you first climb a flight of stairs and are winded, the response is low. When you repeat the stairs and are climbing them easily, you have increased fitness and organ reserve. Your muscles, nerves, and heart have changed in response to stress (adaptation). Even your internal organs will change to adapt to their use or disuse.

You can lose your organ reserve by allowing stress to overwhelm the body until the response becomes inadequate. The healthy person remains healthy because of proper adaptation and function. The person who suffers disease and exhaustion has not adapted and can be truly overwhelmed. Think of a time when you were healthy and happy. Usually it was a time when you had a young physiology with great organ reserve. At other times, when you were exhausted and malnourished, organ reserve was low, and you were easily somewhat depressed, as well as physically sick. Inactivity from a sedentary lifestyle and poor nutrition from consuming processed foods will destroy organ reserve.

Body composition changes with organ reserve. When you're healthy, with a large reserve, you tend to have more active tissue mass (muscle, nerve, bone, visceral organs). With more active tissue, you also tend to stimulate the production of larger, more efficient and more numerous fuel cells (i.e., your mitochondrion). When your body is in a situation where it has to respond by producing energy, it will do the best that it can. Your physical response will usually include an increase in heart rate, respiration, nerve, and muscle activity. This response may not be so effective in the early stages of exercise, especially if you have been inactive. However, if the exercise is not overdone, the body will adapt itself to be able to respond more efficiently in the future. Your body responded with adaptation, or an actual physical change in body structures and capabilities. This is often referred to as the training effect, and it automatically creates more organ reserve.

As you use your body, it begins to change physically in response to the activity. We all know that with the proper exercise, there can be quite a change in physical appearance. Muscles grow in size, and they become more powerful and defined. Stored fat reduces in amount and changes its location of deposition. Bone strengthens, going through structural changes much more important than simply bone mineral density. Tendons, ligaments, and even your internal organs begin to alter in size and improved function. Skin functions and looks better in response. One of the most important changes is the increase in mitochondrial size. The tiny power plants in your cell, the mitochondria, begin to enlarge, become more efficient, and increase the total energy production. Your body can actually work optimally now that it has the energy to do so.

The body is also exposed to the stresses through foreign substances from the environment. We are exposed to pollutants, allergens, insects, pathogens, and chemicals constantly. Some of these are kept out of the body; however, many do gain entrance into the body. When foreign objects are introduced into the body, they create a stress and then your body must mount a response. The detection and response is the responsibility of your immune system. The human body does not make mistakes; it is only doing what it was designed to do. Your body is never doing something wrong; it is always attempting to respond to your lifestyle and the environment to which you subject yourself. First there is a "stressor," and then there is a mechanism for response to that trigger. Your body is just doing its best to keep up with you, and it can be easily overwhelmed if we plan incorrectly or do not plan at all.

There are mental stresses that we are all aware of. It is interesting that mental stresses and physical stresses tend to produce similar responses within the body. You can imagine a stress, such as running away from an elephant who is charging, or you can actually be running from an elephant who is chasing you. In either case, the physiological response can actually be the same. This is true even if you are simply sitting in a chair and it's all playing out in your head. Any stress, real or imagined, calls for a physical response as your body attempts to maintain "homeostasis" or balance. Your body pays constant attention to feedback from its systems, and it does all it can to restore balance when it perceives an imbalance. When we experience stress, there should be some kind of response if everything is working correctly.

Homeostasis is much like a thermostat in a room controlling the air-conditioning system in an attempt to maintain a temperature that you set on the dial. The human body utilizes numerous set points and relies on what we call "negative feedback" and feed forward loops to determine the appropriate response. Your body, as it tries to maintain certain set points, may stimulate systems into action; release hormones, neurotransmitters, or kinases, or send a signal through the nervous system to bring the body back into balance. This may entail stopping some responses as well. The body has many ways in fact to restore balance and return to homeostasis. It is a complicated system, since we are talking about numerous set points adjusting to each other all the same time. How you live your life has the greatest influence on the set points, how your body is operated, and your recovery.

Since stress is unavoidable, the real key is learning how to distinguish good stress or "eustress" from bad stress or "distress." Think about the character Don Quixote, chasing windmills and fighting what would seem to us as insignificant battles. Of course, in his mind these battles were important and justified. This might even have a positive impact on Sir Quixote's psychology. It is of course advantageous to us to possess good judgment about what stress battles are beneficial to us. I submit to you that it is better to devote your time and talents to something that you can actually make a difference in and have a positive impact. Why not follow the advice in Reinhold Niebuhr's serenity prayer: "Grant me the serenity to accept the things I cannot change, the courage to change the things

I can, and the wisdom to know the difference"? There is a lot of stress and response required to chase windmills. Just be sure that the fight is a necessary objective of your life's passion.

Let's revisit the state of "sympathetic dominance." Your sympathetic nervous system is only one part of the autonomic nervous system. There are actually two major divisions of that part of your nervous system that is not voluntary. Remember that breathing and exercise recovery are examples of something that you can do voluntarily, but that are also controlled by the autonomic system. The sympathetic nervous system produces your ability to mount and sustain your fight or flight response. This response is necessary even to be motivated or productive in all aspects of your life. The sympathetic system keeps you physically capable for activities, and maintains your body in a state of readiness for action. There are certain hormones and neural chemicals that are produced when the sympathetic system is activated. Your whole physiology is altered so that you are ready for action. Digestion, sleep, and reproduction, along with recovery and repair systems, are shut down and unavailable until the need for response is over. In fact, upon running the sympathetic system too chronically, the body will actually shut down fat metabolism, and this can drastically affect your ability to maintain your weight.

The parasympathetic system is what facilitates rest and recovery for the body. This is every bit as important, and you need both systems in balance to be healthy. Your parasympathetic system controls sleep, digestion, elimination, and even sexual activity. However, there are many people who spend their time in one system predominately over the other. If you are sympathetic dominant, then you are someone who is always on, and you are continually stimulating your body to be in action mode. If you are using primarily your sympathetic system, then you eventually end up in a state of exhaustion, with all your resources and reserves depleted. If you spend too much of your time utilizing the parasympathetic system, then you are hard pressed to just get things done. You end up sleeping too much, eating too much, and you are unmotivated, even unable to act or react appropriately in situations where you need to.

When designing your state of health, the plan must include striving for a state of balance. Balance would essentially translate to spending time in a parasympathetic state and time in a sympathetic state. The sympathetic system raises your heart rate, blood pressure, respiration, sweating, vision, hearing, and all the things required to take action when there is a threat, or any stress. The parasympathetic system allows for digestion and absorption of nutrients; bowel movements; restoration of hormones, neurotransmitters, and other necessary molecules; sexual activity; sleep; and other functions required for replenishment, rehabilitation, and recovery.

Dr. Robert Sapolsky at Stanford University has studied stress for many years, and he has concluded as a result of his research that the problems with stress occur when the stress is ongoing or nonstop (sympathetic dominant). Dr. Sapolsky studied animals in the wild, in contrast to animals in reserves or protected environments, where the stress is more social. The animals (more frequently in the wild) who are stressed, but then take some physical action (either fight or flight), do not appear to suffer physical damage as a result of their normal stress response. Animals who are protected from predators and have sufficient food available are stressed more by each other, and they do not tend to be as physically active. Dr. Sapolsky believes that they are a perfect model for modern people in society.

Dr. Sapolsky discovered that the animals who experience stress on an ongoing basis, and who do not respond with a physical response such as running away, do experience lasting physical damage. His research shows evidence of dysregulation in the animals' body, especially when it comes to glucose utilization. He has also observed damage to the animal's brain and nervous system---Perhaps even evidence of diseases such as Alzheimer's occurring from stress damage when there is no recovery. When there is no physical activity response, and especially no "down time," the stress response itself becomes dangerous to the animal body, even more than the stressor itself. If the physical response is never carried out, then it would be somewhat like continuing to rev up the engine in your vehicle with the brakes applied. Eventually something will come apart or sustain damage.

Human beings, just like other animals, may not respond appropriately, or let down. Therefore we never alleviate the impact of the stress and the physiological responses produced in our bodies. If the stress response and this alteration of physical chemistry linger for too long, then the stress response itself begins to create physical damage. There is damage to both your physical structure and interference in how well you function. This effect on the nervous system, as well as other biological systems, occurs because the stress response is constantly being triggered. When a zebra in the wild realizes that it is the target of a hungry lioness, then the perceived stress acts as a trigger. The zebra, to facilitate saving its own life, will experience the physiological stress response that prepares the animal for action. This allows the zebra have a chance to be successful, allowing it to react quickly and effectively enough to get away from the lion, and perhaps even defend itself with a well-placed kick.

The lion, who will die without feeding on a regular basis, is also under stress that will trigger physiological changes. The lion must be in this ready state or risk missing the kill—and starvation. In the case of both animals, if there is physical response, then their bodies are not damaged as a result of the stress. Each animal will then have some recovery time to be prepared for the next situation or opportunity. The only real problem is whether the lioness will eat, or the zebra will live. It is not a question of the danger of stress itself. Exercise has the advantage of creating a sympathetic response as you perform a physical activity. Exercise also has the benefit of a reflex response from the parasympathetic system. You warm up and exercise with intensity because your body responded to allow this. Then, as soon as you stop exercising, your body will automatically shift to the parasympathetic system so that you can recover.

In human beings, at least in modern society, we retain the fight or flight response to any stress, but it is not often acted upon. In fact, many people remain in that "turned on" state for every hour of every day. Some of us seem to be in that state constantly for most of our lives. I am saying that if those people when stressed would be physically active, they would alleviate the potential for physical harm to themselves. We see people all the time who are negatively impacted by stress and have concluded that the only response is to tolerate the stress. Remember, in nature the body makes ready for a response, and then there is a response. If there is no actual physical response, only the body making ready for a response, this is sympathetic dominance.

If we are to learn to use stress for adaptation, then we have to look no further than the science called *allostasis*. The allostatic load is the sum of all the stresses applied to your body and to your mind. If your body can mount an adequate response, it will lead to either a positive adaptation, or a negative maladaptation. The human body never makes a mistake; it is only attempting to keep up with your lifestyle. If the stress is overwhelming or is too repetitive, then the response will be more difficult to recover from. However, if you are adapting correctly, then each time the stress appears, your response will lessen as your body becomes more prepared. This is adaptation.

That is why physical therapists and scientists study allostasis. When you're referred to see a physical therapist, perhaps to recover from a knee injury, allostatic load is considered. The therapist will design a stretching and exercise routine that will carefully and strategically apply stresses to your knee. It may be painful, and the work is done with great effort on your part and the therapist's part. But if allostasis is applied correctly, then you will very possibly end up with a knee that is stronger and more stable than ever before—this in many cases without any surgical intervention. Your knee adapted in response to the stress, all according to the plan of the physical therapist. We benefit if we find a way to control the force, which is stress.

Chapter 14

Motivation and Success

Here we are near the end of this book, and I am sure that you have started to formulate a plan. I believe that you will even implement your plan, but I cannot stop here until I give you reason to continue on.

I am part of a very effective program in our clinic. We have been witness to miraculous changes in peoples' lives as they get off medications, restore vitality, and literally live in a new body after twelve weeks. I mean that diseases that they had thought would be with them for the rest of their lives have been resolved. At that point, the difficulty is to maintain good health and, better yet, continue to improve their state of wellness. When you are accountable within a program you have committed to, you can stick with it, especially if you see results and feel better. Now as you take over the management of your lifestyle, life happens. Financial pressure, kids, relatives, jobs, schedules, injury, and traumas are part of life can take us off track. If you get too far off track, it is easy to rely on old habits that did not work before, but it is all we feel we can do. How can we all stay motivated in the heat of the struggle?

It is now more evident to you just how much of a part that you play in the creation of either wellness or chronic disease. You can quite possibly prevent disease from ever occurring in the first place, as long as you don't allow an internal environment that would promote it. We used to believe that genetics and your family history were predetermined fates for you to live out. Unfortunately, some still believe that prevention is only finding a problem or disease process early enough to be able to slow its progression. Many practitioners still believe that if your parents experienced a certain disease, you should simply resign yourself to dealing with the same disease. Too often the plan is to wait until the disease is advanced enough, and then treatment can begin. The old concept is that if something existed in your genes, you were now susceptible to that disease process, and somehow you were given unlucky genetics. Genetic expression was thought of as nothing more than the expected outcome.

Designing a Congruent Lifestyle

I prefer to think of your DNA as an elegant record of how your ancestors survived. Everything that they did to adapt to their environment is recorded in your genes. This allowed your ancestors to be successful, while others failed to thrive, so that eventually your parents could be here and produce you. Programmed into your genes are their stress responses (genetic expressions) that were necessary at the time, and which still could be beneficial today. To the contrary, some of their responses and genetic annotations might create dysfunctions or even disease in your current situation. It is exactly like opening a comprehensive reference book and searching for a solution that worked well in the past. You may determine that it is exactly the right response today, as it was in the past. You might also realize that the previous solution might lead to more problems in modern times. You may also have to change the way that you do things, knowing the information.

Your DNA contains information that you use constantly. Some parts are blueprints or representations for something that your body needs to develop, manufacture, or regenerate. Other references may induce processes that are not required or may even be detrimental. Your genetic expression comes down to the results of your body referencing your DNA to contend with the situations you have created in your life. Your total living environment may also have to be tailored to situations that your body can handle in a positive way with the right information. It is all about finding the proper environment for you to live in, which matches your choices for nutrition, physical activity, and whatever you expose your body to. Your DNA is packed with information concerning what to do and how to react to environmental situations. If you learn the environment that fits your genes best, and then live according to that knowledge, you will feel great and look better than you ever thought possible.

Life itself, and keeping your physical body healthy in the midst of it, is a dynamic and ongoing project. Your ancestors lived their lives and had their experiences, which they chemically marked in your DNA. It's as if they gave you a journal of their life that you might be able to benefit from in yours. If you look away for even a moment, the concept of time will still move forward without you. It takes a fair amount of motivation to focus on and participate in a healthy lifestyle that is congruent with how your body can perform.

Stay Motivated, or Abandon Your Health?

It is very easy to talk about doing something, but actually getting it done creates the magic. I am not telling you anything that you don't already know here. Some people can be self-motivated if they just understand that there will be enough of a payoff. Others need to be pushed, prodded, and cajoled, and they will still wait until last possible moment to take action before it's too late. We are all aware that the payoff comes in the form of good health. Be reminded that once you let your health go, it can be very difficult to get it back. I am suggesting that you reprioritize your health.

When I say I will "try" to be healthy, I can put it off until some other time. For something to happen, you have to do it now, in the present. If you are not self-motivated to maintain your health, and you need a little push, then consider the fact that the quality of your life is literally up to you. This is not condescending or patronizing, since I absolutely believe that it is within your power to be healthy and experience wellness. It is important to ask yourself whether you want to actively participate in life, or whether you want to be the inactive bystander, perhaps eventually using some assistive device? It is a choice that you make every single day. I point this out only because so many people have come to believe that their health is in the hands of a doctor or some other practitioner. Religious or spiritual faith are absolutely important, but when it comes to your health, how you live your life determines your results. We know now that health is an ongoing process, and it is a response, and absolutely not simply a predetermined fate.

One of my passions is to inspire people to focus more upon their current state of health, and then to see them actually realize their true health potential. I want everyone to learn and use any tool at their disposal that will keep them living at an optimal level, not simply sustaining their lives. It is my dream to help people minimize their need for the use of medication. I love designing strategies that help people to discover available, effective alternatives to medication, until they can reach the self-sufficiency that comes from being healthy. I am also passionate about showing people what real food actually is and helping them understand the dangers created when we consume industrialized and processed food. Your health is my passion, every bit as much as my own state of health. I have seen enough evidence that there is a better way than simply waiting around to get sick and then seeking a treatment.

The Creation of Effective Motivation

What are your passions? I encourage you to ask, and then answer, this question for yourself. Most people simply cannot come up with a good answer to this question because they have not taken the time to even consider it. Some of us have answered this question in the past, but time passes, and our passions might change as well. Others had passions but have lost focus on them as they went about life. A few people have never even had a passion at all. I am not talking about a passionate relationship, or even a sexual encounter. I am asking you to capture your core beliefs, and the passion that drives you and makes life worth living. This is not about your children, your family, or your job; it is about your paradigm.

A paradigm is a pattern, or model of hypothesis, in science. It is also our judgment of what is real and how things work. You have your beliefs and judgment that cannot be challenged easily or shaken. You are "passionate" about them, and you will defend them and desire them. Do you know absolutely what your passions are, or have you been just living day to day and getting by? Again, this is not a simple list of dreams or musings; I am talking about the things that you will live and die for. What are your passions? I want you to be on track and in line with all the things that are really important to you. Just because they are important to *you*. "World peace," or a "clean environment" sound real nice, but if they don't exist as a gut feeling for you, then I encourage you to look a little deeper.

It has been said that "there are many things in life that will catch your eye, but only a few things will catch your heart." Pursue those things. Your passions are those things you carry that are deeply embedded in who you are. You can be passionate about many things; however, your true core passions usually number only a few. These are the people, objects, or ideals that are most important to your being. These are the things that make your life worth living. These are the things that you're ultimately here to accomplish. Your life will not be fulfilled until you have discovered what these things are and become set on a path toward their completion.

If you don't know your own passions, there are probably people around you who do know them. Someone close to you who can "press your buttons" and get a reaction from you. They have observed what is important to you, and they use it because they know you will rise to its defense. Think about what makes you stand up in defense, or take the leap. Many people who identify what they are passionate about abandon that passion in favor of something else that they believe "needs" to be done. But if you're not living your dreams, you are living and working toward someone else's passion. It's hard to imagine committing to live your life with someone and not even to be aware of what they are passionate about. However, it is very common for people to plan a life together, even consider marriage or legal partnership, and really have not the slightest idea as to what their partner's real dreams are. It is very easy to state dreams that sound good to others, but are they your true passions?

I am discussing this subject of passions because, if and when you identify your passion, then you have the most effective tool that there is for self-motivation. When you can visualize your dreams, and realize that you are on track toward your passion, then you are motivated, and it becomes nearly impossible to stop or dissuade you. Detours can be permanent, or they can be only temporary. We have to keep focus on our destination, always knowing the compass bearing even if we have to change course. As long as we know our destination, even after a detour, we can reset our course. I know this seems self-evident to you, but I bring it up because so many people literally stuff their passions out of sight, only to find them later and regret the fact that they missed their destination. The dreams that are really important to you I hope will not be forgotten.

Often other people know your passions because you won't stop talking about them. When you are focused, you create the motivation, and you pick up momentum. When you share passions and dreams with other people, they can read your excitement and your commitment. Share dreams with enough people, and you will find things start happening even faster, as there is strength in numbers. It is very easy to ignore what is important to you and then lose the passion by getting busy in day-to-day life. It is just like placing your dreams in a shoebox under the bed, only to open the box years later and experience regret. This while others who kept focused and motivated ended up with exactly what they wanted.

"If I Knew I Was Going to Live This Long, I'd Have Taken Better Care of Myself"

Research has demonstrated that living with regrets will not only reduce your quality of life; it will shorten your life. I encourage you to let go of regrets, re-identify your dreams today, and take your first step. Some of us need motivation outside of ourselves, while others are continually self-motivated. The strategy then is to figure out what works best for us to produce motivation, and then put it to use. If you need motivation from outside of yourself, I encourage you to find tools for the motivation and use them effectively. You may have to look at things in a whole different way and reconstruct your priorities. Even if it is against all the odds—if it is your passion, pursue it. When you know your passion, your real dream for life, you have the greatest tool available to be motivated.

The most common thing that I see people lose motivation for is exercise. Yet I know of no better tool to rebuild the body to create optimum function and health. I also believe that exercise is an important component of practically anyone's passion. Let's analyze this a little further. It will be difficult to live well and experience any passion, or even see it fulfilled, without your body functioning in good health. One of the most common regrets quoted, as someone nears the end of their life, is the lack of health. How many times have you heard the saying, "I wish I'd taken better care of myself"? We all want to live long; however, it is quality of life that I believe everyone is looking for.

If your objective is to participate fully in life, then it will require a certain level of physical function and health. Physical exercise keeps all the biological systems of the body switched on and functioning. Lack of activity allows the body to shut down and become dysfunctional. If we do stay on task to take better care of ourselves, then we will enjoy our passions without that regret. What good is a lifetime of accomplishments if we don't have the health to enjoy them? Keeping this in mind develops more motivation, seeking the results that the physical activity will produce. If you want these results to last for your lifetime, you must motivate and empower yourself and stay consistent. If you can build motivation for consistent physical activity, you also empower your drive for your dreams.

Definition of Motivation

We define things to better understand them, so that we can use them. *Motivation* is defined in textbooks as an internal state or condition that activates behavior and gives it direction; motivation is a desire or want that energizes and directs goal-oriented behavior; motivation is the influence of perceived needs and desires on the intensity and direction of behavior. Franken (1994) provides an additional component in his definition: "motivation being the arousal, direction, and persistence of behavior." To realize a goal, we must take consistent action to move toward it and, at the same time, keep focus on the desired end result. This does not mean that we cannot enjoy the journey and get what we want at the same time.

While still not widespread in terms of introductory psychology textbooks, many researchers are now beginning to acknowledge that the factors that energize behavior are likely different from the factors that provide for its persistence. No matter what starts you on the path to your dreams, there is also the need to constantly revisit your reasoning. We must be ready to evaluate when we are off track and make adjustments as necessary. For several years, I worked aboard ships going to sea. When orders came to carry a cargo to a certain destination, it was expected that we would reach that place in a safe and timely manner with our product. This required more than simply pointing the ship in the right direction as we left our home port and hope things turned out. We were expected to deliver the cargo and not give up or get distracted.

Aboard the ship, before departing, it was necessary to consult charts and books and computers. We needed to check the weather and currents presently, and then the conditions expected in the future during the voyage. We had to be especially prepared for any problems should they arise by stocking the right supplies, inspecting equipment, and checking our safety gear. After all, we might be far out to sea and need to take care of a problem on our own. We would actually draw a line on the chart, showing where we wanted to go and allowing us to make accurate estimates on how long it might take, and if we were traveling along the best route. Many people would consult the chart during our trip, and knowing the plan help keep us moving toward the expected result.

However, the ship was not often right on top of that line drawn on the chart. Constant adjustments were made in steering, and the ship's course would be changed—sometimes a little, and other times radically. At times, we did not know exactly where we were; however, we could use a process referred to as "dead reckoning" and anticipate our position. At the next opportunity, we could get a "fix" on our position, and because we were focused on our destination and monitoring our progress, most of the time our anticipated position and our real position remained close. Some things could be anticipated on our journey, while other problems, while unplanned, would cause a deviation. But with ongoing corrections, we made it every time.

If we consult psychology textbooks, we might read that motivation is a reason or set of reasons for engaging in a particular behavior. Human behavior is extensively studied in psychology and neuropsychology. The reason for persistence in a behavior seems to include our basic needs (e.g., food, water, shelter). We will also persist in a behavior to obtain an object, goal, state of being, or ideal that is desirable. If the goal we persist toward is viewed as "positive," our basic motivation can be defined as pleasure. At least we are seeking a state of being in which pain is absent. The motivation for behavior may also be attributed to less-apparent reasons, such as altruism or morality. Regardless of the reason for the motivation, that thing that we want is regarded as a necessity, since it is incorporated into our purpose and reason for living.

The Strategy of Motivation

There are a number of suggested strategies to creating motivation. If you talk to yourself the way you would talk to someone that you love or care about, you can create more effective motivation. "Self-talk" is defined in many practices, such as neurolinguistic programming (NLP). Many researchers have discovered that your brain is indeed plastic and programmable. You can indeed reinforce the structure and programming of your brain by talking to yourself. This talk must be positive in order to keep motivation alive. When you tell yourself that you cannot do something, then you will facilitate not being able to do it.

I recall a good illustration of this in the movie titled *The Edge*. This is a movie about three men being hunted by a bear in the Alaskan wilderness. The bear is intent on killing the men after smelling and tasting the blood of one of the trio. They are losing hope since they do not see any way to defend themselves, and the bear will not stop its pursuit. It seems the bear might win. Then, the actor Anthony Hopkins, who plays one of the characters, pulls out a matchbox cover depicting a picture of an Indian killing a bear with a wooden pole. He turns to his companion and states, "What one man can do, another can do. We are going to kill the bear." See the movie to watch what happens. Believing in yourself is the most important part of motivation—and success.

Motivation Made Simple

I will finish this chapter with a less complicated but very resonant discussion about motivation. If we break motivation down to its bare essentials, then we can look at what really motivates all of us. Motivation is essentially produced by either pain or pleasure. In fact, I suggest that we illustrate the concept of motivation in terms of either a carrot or a stick. The horse pulling a carriage can be motivated to pull the cart by holding a carrot out in front, where the horse can perceive that it can move closer and then enjoy eating the carrot. We can also get that horse to move by hitting it with a stick or a whip. The horse then perceives that if it does not move forward, there will be more pain.

Furthermore, if I am motivated to move toward a carrot as my reward, I become proactive in pressing forward. If I seek pleasure as my motivation, I think about moving toward the "carrot," or something I am passionate about. I have focused on a result, and I have a plan to keep moving forward. If I am motivated by pain, on the other hand, I will tend to wait until the pain is more than I can bear before I take any action. Only when I feel that I can't take it anymore am I motivated to do something about it. At this point there is no plan or goal—just a need to stop the pain. As soon as the pain is minimized, then progress stops, and I wait for the next time that pain is unbearable. This cycle of pain-aversion-pain will get you through life, but what kind of life is that?

I am reminded of two quarter horse breeding and training facilities that I was acquainted with a few years ago. There are two ranches not that far from each other in distance, but their way of thinking was actually worlds apart. On one ranch, domination, or establishing the trainer as the alpha, was the key to training. To prove that you are the lead and dominant animal, the other animals must actually anticipate your reprisal if they displease you. This method relies on fear, and possibly pain, if you do not know your place or perform as desired by the leader. The alpha, in this case the trainer, figuratively carried a huge "stick."

On this particular ranch, spurs were worn and used often, whips were cracking, and horses would be hobbled or tied to posts, basically made to succumb to the wish of the trainer or rider. This ranch produced excellent horses that were ready for gathering cows and working the ranch, as well as being ready for competition-level performance. The owner of this ranch had many ribbons and awards for his horses, and he was very respected as a horse trainer and competitor. In fact, every animal that he owned understood his dominance and treated him like the alpha. He demanded respect, and every animal knew its place. Any animal that did not fall into line would experience the pain that accompanied disobedience.

At the other ranch, things just seemed more relaxed. This trainer used praise and patience for what is today referred to as positive reinforcement training. There were no spurs used, or whips, or hobbles. The horses were never force-tied for training or "breaking"; in fact, they were taught to not fight the lead rope, but to simply follow it. Blood was never drawn during training, and the animals on this ranch did not know pain (or a stick) as a training device. However, the horses from this ranch were also champions, and this owner had as many trophies and ribbons. The animals on this ranch seemed willing to do anything to please the trainer, and receive his praise.

They took pleasure in the possibility of doing well, and they even seemed to enjoy a crowd of onlookers, being quite taken with themselves. They seemed to know that they were good, or at least that they had done something right. Horses from both ranches learned to respond to the lightest touch of any rider, which is a desirable trait. However, horses from the first ranch would read their rider and respond to avoid anticipated pain. Horses from the second ranch wanted the pleasure of listening to and pleasing the rider. I hope that we all live more in a world where we receive praise, instead of one where we constantly run from pain.

Most modern animal trainers have found that the positive reinforcement of behaviors is much more productive than any other style of training. Animals and humans respond in a very similar manner. Think about designing a lifestyle where you are proactive and moving forward to receive pleasure. Modern-day medicine is really much more like the first ranch. When it comes to our health, most people are not doing a lot of things that I would consider proactive. Strategies such as eating nutritionally sound food and being physically active could be likened to seeking a carrot, but they could also be avoiding the stick. Generally people don't do much about their health or consult a physician until they have a health problem and things have gone wrong. May people will wait until that problem is fairly serious. In our current system, the physician is trained to identify disease and render a diagnosis, both big sticks.

Once the diagnosis is made, there is an appropriate treatment administered, which may last for an extended period of time. There is no end in sight, just management of the disease. There is not even any discussion about fixing the problem, only managing it with ongoing treatment. In a way, the more important health or function issue is ignored, and the disease is left in place, allowing it to develop further. Often, as time goes by, the situation grows more serious (the stick gets bigger), and people are motivated to return for more treatment. In this scenario, there is no understanding of function or patterns, just identification of symptoms. There is no strategy except to return to the practitioner when your problem recurs or develops. Our system is based on palliative care only until the next stick appears. When you are avoiding sticks, the only plan is to get away from the stick.

I recommend going all out for the carrot. Honestly, if you are taking care of yourself properly, you can completely avoid the stick. When you keep your body functioning well, you don't allow disease to even start. I have observed that you cannot even gain excess weight. In fact, it will be rare that you even experience the pain, or the stick, because you are proactive. When you have your goal in sight, and you are planning something ahead, you end up even anticipating how to move forward more effectively. You are proactive, and you actually prevented the serious problem before it could start, let alone become serious. You never allowed an environment to be created in your body that would even allow disease. Prevention is best defined as never experiencing a problem. In the words of an old desert navigator, "Fix a point on the horizon and steer by that point."

Steps to Success: Formulate The Plan

I really do want you all to be successful and to enjoy success with good health and vitality. I strongly believe that everyone has it within their own power to live a life ruled by wellness and optimum quality. Of course, there are some people who have been presented with more challenges than others. However, if there is a plan or strategy in place, every person can at the very minimum improve upon their situation. I have discussed throughout this book the concept of being proactive instead of reactive. Proactive people refuse to accept the status quo, especially in their own life situations. When anyone tells you that there is nothing that can be done, and that you must live with your current status, then I suggest that you find someone better to listen to. You do not have to accept things the way they are. Opinions vary, and no matter what authority tells you to lie down and give up, you can always find a second opinion. If we think it out and explore ideas together, formulate strategies, create modifications, and search the trails, the way will be discovered.

I fully understand that one must be realistic, but that does not mean that we abandon all hope. No one knows what you can accomplish or are capable of, once you have set your mind to do it. For example, let us say that you see one surgical "expert" who tells you that you have no choice but to have surgery, and that this will place severe limitations upon what you can do. I suggest that you look for another surgeon who has seen more success with their patients. I am reminded of a patient who I was working with years ago. He had a very debilitating accident. He was told that he needed a surgery which would be extensive, extremely risky, and invasive. He was also told that he probably would never walk again and to be prepared for life in a wheelchair. He decided not to accept this scenario. Instead he found a different surgeon, another authority, who would work with him and who had a more positive outlook. He opted to try physical rehabilitation first to at least improve the success of any surgery. The exercise therapy was successful enough that he avoided all but a minor surgical procedure. In fact, he was so determined that he continued to push himself beyond expectations. He later returned to compete in triathlons, which were his passion. He did not focus on limitations; he focused on the possibilities.

The Limitations Are in Your Mind

There is no one who can claim to know exactly where your ceiling of achievement is, or how limited you will be. Only you can test your boundaries and truly understand your limits. How do you really know whether you can do something, or how well you can actually perform, unless you make the attempt? Much of the time, the only limitations are in your own mind. People often surprise themselves, and others around them, when they challenge themselves as far as they can. Of course, the challenge can be overwhelming, and many times it has to be broken up into small steps with modifications. However, if we never make the attempt to improve beyond perceived limitations, I guarantee you that something will be missed.

In my opinion, there are too many people who seem to accept physical disability as a way of life. There are programs successfully getting people out of bed, out of wheelchairs, and free from walkers. There are studies of people at virtually any age utilizing exercise to regain the mobility they had when they were younger. When it comes to your health, don't let anyone tell you that you need to give up or give in. The human body has a fantastic capacity for rehabilitation. You can get stronger, you can improve balance, and you can reduce disability.

How can you understand what your limitations are until you experiment and test it out for yourself? Of course, reference information and confer with other authorities who may have even better strategies that allow you to rise above or dance beyond these perceived limitations. The only honest answer a practitioner can give to you would be, "I don't know what your limits really are. I don't know how long you have to live. I really don't know what you could be capable of, and in my experience this is what I have seen under similar circumstances." Sometimes it is worth seeking out people who have knowledge of better experiences and outcomes. We are talking about *you* here—your body, your mind, and your quality of life. I implore you not to simply accept what you're told without question. This is something that you need to know for yourself.

I had a patient who had some minor back pain and decided that he would undergo surgery to relieve it. The surgeon promised and insisted that this procedure would solve all the problems. This surgeon further recommended that the patient would be better off with a metal cage placed between two vertebra for more stability. This young man had a promising career in sports and was likely to go from college to the NFL. The surgery was not as successful as promised, and this young man ended up suffering with even more extensive pain. The same surgeon who had promised that after surgery the patient would be able to play professional football now advised the young man not to pursue any sports career. The doctor said, furthermore, that the best thing this young man could do would be to limit any physical activity and just live with the pain. The young man was told to be careful doing any lifting, running, or, for that matter, anything physical involving his back. The young man felt as if his life was over and, along with the acceptance of more pain, sank into depression, quit school, and was destined for lifelong disability.

However, there is a positive turn to the story. Two years later, he met an athletic trainer who had experience with post-surgical rehabilitation. He also returned to our clinic for chiropractic treatment. As he started to feel slightly better, the young man decided to test his limits and see for himself what he was really capable of doing. It was not long before he was out of pain and had himself created the necessary strength and stability in his lower back by properly rehabilitating the muscles and ligaments of his lower back. It was not long after this that he was able to stop using the pain medication and was off all the antidepressants. I don't know that he ever was able to play football again, but I do know that by not accepting limits, he explored his potential and found himself much better off. You see, the athletic trainer and I had seen the possibility and the potential in this man, because in our experience, we had seen others overcome their limitations. The reason that this story ends well is solely because of the resolve of the young man.

When anyone tells you that you must accept a life of limitation, that is just their opinion, which is based only on their experience. Whether it is a physician, some other professional authority, or your best friend, it is only their opinion. You don't have to accept it, and I recommend that you explore all the possibilities for yourself. Another acquaintance of mine lives in the northeastern United States in a very beautiful home. He has excelled in life by most standards not because he believes he is more intelligent or gifted, but because he enjoys rising to a challenge. Whenever someone tells him that something cannot be done, his passion becomes finding a way to prove them wrong. He finds a way to get the "impossible" done, and this has made him a very rich man. We all need to be careful about accepting poor health or disability as aging or some expected disease phenomenon. When people focus on living a lifestyle that embraces better function, many things seem to improve. If we understand that every problem has a mechanism, we can study that mechanism and then find way to improve or even eliminate the problem. Whether it is allergies, autoimmune disease, heart disease, or simply a recurring headache, there is an answer which can be found.

How to Write the Plan

The responsibility for fulfilling your passions in life rests squarely on your shoulders. I do hope that one of your passions is wellness, or at least includes health. Fulfillment does not just happen; it begins with a plan. Everybody has a plan at least to take the first step, or perhaps a plan to wait and see. The fighter Joe Louis is quoted as saying, "Everyone has a plan, until they've been hit." A good plan still functions even after you have been hit. I mentioned earlier that when working aboard a ship, everything was planned and executed to get the job done. When it was time to proceed to the next port, the course we would take had to be drawn right on the chart. That line on the chart would be followed, even though adjustments were required all along the way to stay close to that line. The line was a plan. There was a plan for everything that you've ever done successfully. Flying by the seat of your pants and trusting luck can work out for you, but even this started with some sort of a plan. Luck doesn't always tend to be reliable; plans and contingency adjustments work much more consistently.

If you want to make something happen, then there are certain steps that we all know we must take. The first step is knowing your objective with at least the concept of a plan. If you don't even know where it is you want to go, you live a life filled with random destinations. These destinations will likely have nothing to do with what you are passionate about. Wandering can be exciting, but at the same time it might just waste too much of your precious time. There are many writings and discussions about the concept of creating your own reality. Your current reality, or your paradigm, contains all your beliefs and all your judgments about what is possible and what is not. Your paradigm is what is "real" to you. I want you to consider that you can develop your paradigm, or your truth, and include everything that you really want in this reality that is yours. I want for you good health, plenty of energy and vitality, and the freedom created by wellness. If you placed that in your paradigm as one goal, it complements everything else. Creating reality includes realizing new dreams and possessing what it is that we really want.

Initially, though, we have to know what it is that we want. It is interesting to me that when you ask most people what it is that they really want, they don't have an answer. Sure, we can all wax dreamy and talk about things that would be "nice" or "fun" or that "sound good," but are these really what we want? The majority of people are so involved in their day-to-day lives that they have lost sight of anything that they really desire. Try sitting down and writing a list of your goals, dreams, aspirations, and things that you have a desire for. Don't let there be any constraints for that list. This initial list is not to be judged by money, time, your resources, or your abilities; it is a list of possibilities that you want to create. First, understand what it is that you hope for; then you can move toward what you actually want. Hope is where people get stalled, because hope without taking action is simply hoping for the best that may never come.

If you can generate a real and comprehensive list in just a few minutes, then you are among the minority of people who know what they want. You are also likely on your way to getting it. However, if you have to contemplate, stare at the ceiling, or struggle to think of anything meaningful, then I believe you are off track and your life is not congruent with what you want. When you can focus on what is most important to you, then you begin to see it formulate and finally appear before your eyes. When you are focused on your dream, you will see possibilities and opportunities that you would have otherwise missed completely. You might not know where to start, or perhaps you know the first three steps of a hundred steps needed for completion. When you focus on the goal, your own mind is working around the clock on solutions, and the steps become clear, just like completing a jigsaw puzzle. How can you take advantage of opportunities that you're unaware of?

Keep a paper and pen within your reach at night, and especially when you awaken. Many problems have been solved or steps toward a goal discovered during sleep, which you can record and not forget about. Perhaps you will encounter someone who has the know-how or the resources that will help you. Since you were thinking about your goal, this opportunity for help was not missed. There are a multitude of stories of people who are only too happy to help others attain a dream. When you are focused and intent on your passion, or even some need, other people pick that up. They may even step up and provide your whole solution. I know of a couple who heard of someone who needed somewhere to live as a result of a foreclosure on their home. This couple had the ability and resources to purchase a house and then provided it because they had asked. There are so many people who love to help others, whether they can give you a house or perhaps just give you a hand. However, if they are not aware of your need or your passion because you are not aware of it, nothing will ever happen.

How can so many people not even know what it is that they want? Think of many of the people that you are acquainted with. Consider how they struggle, how they are so busy surviving their life, that they probably don't have much of a plan. Getting through is not a plan, but it is a limited existence. I suggest that the first step to creating a plan is to create a written list of things that we really want. It is not effective to just keep this in your head; writing adds another dimension. Once you begin to focus on your real passions, they begin to take shape and have started to become reality. It is best to review your list every day. The list may be altered, even completely changed, because it is your list. It is imperative that we not lose focus on the things that make up our list.

When you have created your list, is a good idea to filter the items on that list. Look at every item on the list and make sure that you can come up with a good reason for it to be there. What is the "why," or the reason that this item is even on your list? If you can't easily come up with the why, then that item is likely only a whim or a dream that should not be on this list. This is an ongoing exercise to constantly establish what is really important to you. Bringing things into reality starts with giving them existence by creating dimension. For example, if it is a house that you want, create drawings, collect pictures, even build a model of the house, and be very specific. If you want a new car, go sit in a car just like the one you want. Feel it, see it, taste it. First we must know what it is that we want; then we can begin to build the dimensions. It is not long before it is real.

Programming the Plan into Your Mind

There is a concept called "top-of-your-mind awareness." A good indication of your mind's current focus and current priorities is the foremost thought in your mind. If the subjects on the top of your mind are not yours, then they are someone else's priorities. In essence, you are working on somebody else's dream. We all have a tendency toward attention-deficit disorder—that inability to stay focused on what is important to us. Distraction is all around us, and to keep focused on your passions, the only way I know of is to continually make them more real by keeping them in our crosshairs.

Advertisers know how to do this perhaps better than we do ourselves. Think of any product. If the marketing was successful, you can very accurately describe it in all dimensions. Perhaps you have already purchased it and it is sitting at home. Marketers know how your neurology works, and they do everything they can to own that top-of-your-mind thinking. They will create a desire in you by giving dimension to the product and demonstrating the benefits of whatever they are selling. They can get you to take action on things not even that important to you. It is a distraction, or their intention, that becomes your focus.

Human beings receive information from their environment through the senses. Sight (ophthalmoception), hearing (audioception), taste (gustaoception), smell (olfacoception or olfacception), and touch (tactioception) are the five traditionally recognized senses, and the only senses proven to exist in humans. There are also senses that include temperature (thermoception), kinesthetic sense (proprioception), pain (nociception), balance (equilibrioception) and acceleration (kinesthesioception). We use the information gathered from senses to create our paradigm. Interpreting and judging this information is our way of evaluating the world around us.

It creates what we believe to be our truth. We determine what we perceive to be safe or not, to be pain or pleasure, or to be real or fantasy.

We can actually focus so much on some information to the exclusion of other facts that may be important. Often we actually do not even perceive all the facts. This will affect our judgment and perhaps even our reality. For example, have you ever been concentrating so intently on something, and then been startled by someone walking into the room? You did not even see them. There are puzzles that are pictures, and depending on how you focus on the picture, the image will change. Your mind will even try to fill in the blanks for you when you don't have all the information. That is why we all must be careful making assumptions when we have not evaluated all the available information.

Your brain is every bit as programmable as the computer that you likely use every day. Your top-of-mind awareness is the program running at the moment. If you do not find that your priorities are there and opened, then you have stopped working on them. There is an area in your brainstem referred to as the reticular (network) formation. This is where you collect all the data that establishes your paradigm and your reality. All of the information that you can perceive from the environment is filtered through this network formation. When you hear, see, feel, taste, smell, etc., all the information will be selectively evaluated and create or design what you believe to be real.

Just like writing this book, since I am using word-processing software, the software must be running, and this particular document must be open. Otherwise, the book will not get done because it is out of sight and out of mind. Your top-of-mind awareness is all your open documents. Even as we write in a document, we are communicating dimension, giving detail, and making something more real than it was before. The more senses that you can engage, the more real something is. A dream in your head is a concept without much description. The more information that you provide and communicate, the more you give dimension and make it real.

Creating your own reality, then, is continually adding the details and dimensions. When you have a written list that has been filtered by the "why," you have added dimension. Another dimension is priority and time. Where does each item fit in its importance and urgency to you? When does it need to be done, and when do you know that it is complete? Use all of your senses to describe these parameters as well. The fact is that we all give our priorities attention each day. If you don't agree, or if you don't like what you are focused on today, then change the list for tomorrow, because it is worth considering putting your priorities first.

A Life Out of Balance Tips Over

An important concept to develop as well is balance. Categorize each item into a small number of divisions. Is the item for you personally, something you want to own, to be, to do, or even your legacy? Is it about your family, something that primarily applies to them? Is it a goal for your job or something that you are engaged in each day? Is it about a group or an organization like a church or a club? Establish the primary category for each of your true goals. Now I would have you analyze how many items are in each category. If there are numerous personal goals but only one or two for your family, you are on track to lose your family. If many goals are in work, but nothing for yourself, is this really what you want? What about the many women who give everything for the family and are "selfless" and devoted. It is not long before their health suffers and they are in need of care themselves.

The categories that are important to you must be in balance. The person who puts everything into their work, only to realize that life has passed them by and they do not know their family, is a good example of what not to do. They tell themselves that they were doing it for the family, but the next thing that they know, the kids have grown or the family is gone. If they had balanced work priorities with family priorities, they would have been able to enjoy both. If your categories are not in balance, then either add some priorities to the category that is low, or drop some from the overfilled category. Your choice is to either rebalance, or let the less-populated category fall apart.

As your list becomes more real, dimension and description are moving the things you want closer to existence. It is not real until you commit to do it. For anyone with integrity, your signature is your word, and your word is your bond. I encourage you to place your signature next to each goal. Authorize and certify that you're going to do this thing that is important to you. When you sign your name, things change, because instead of simply thinking about it, you have committed to it. I remember a patient of mine who was coming in frequently with back pain and other health complaints. After some time, I spoke with him about actually correcting his problems rather than getting temporary relief and treatment. I talked with him about altering his diet and getting some exercise.

In fact, I told him, there is a 5K race in a few months and I want you to enter. My intention was to get him to prepare for the race and get into better shape. Of course, he was a busy executive, and although he agreed and told me and others he would do something, things really did not change. However, he did sign up for the race, paid money, and literally "signed his name." Race day arrived, and he felt committed, so he actually went to the race unprepared. He was passed by little kids, had to stop several times, and by the time he reached the finish line, no one was there to cheer for him. In fact, the finish line had been taken down, by the time he got there. He was so upset that little kids had passed him that he signed up for another race and began to investigate how to be prepared. This time on race day, he was able to do the entire race without stopping, people cheered him at the finish line, and not one child got by him.

Next thing I know, he was doing a 10K, a half marathon, and then an entire full marathon. He even became a marathon running coach, just to inspire other people. During this time he dropped 120 pounds of fat and muscled up, since he started to feel the benefits from exercise beyond running. He had been eating better to prepare and was motivated by the difference that he felt. Now, with some lifestyle changes, his back pain, joint pain, and muscle pain were non-existent. He no longer experienced allergies, gastroesophageal reflux, or irritable bowel syndrome. The only time I would see him after that is occasionally out in public, since he really didn't need treatment at the clinic. He attributes all of this to the fact that he signed his name, committing to the first 5K race.

I hope that your health is included as a goal in your life's plan. Each day that passes when you don't incorporate positive physical activity is another day that your body degenerates. Every day that you do not focus on good nutrition is another day that your body must perform triage. Life is an ongoing experience, and unfortunately we cannot turn it off and come back to it later. You have to be careful not to change channels and focus on the wrong thing at the expense of something that was important to you. You are part of the recreation of your physical body and your mind every single day you exist. When you're not focused on positive adaptations, then you will end up with a response—but not necessarily of your liking.

Chapter 15

Final Thoughts

It is my dream and it is my passion to inspire you. I am certain that many people who scan through this book, or those who read it word for word, are already familiar with the concept of health. They appreciate, at least intellectually, that wellness is more desirable than illness, and they do appreciate the value of a functional state of being. Dr. Jeffrey Bland, who has been an inspiration to me over the years, talks about people living lives of self-destruction and de-evolution. Evolution should create a beneficial response to our current environment, allowing us to adapt and survive. In the studies of Dr. Bland and other researchers, it has been found that not only is lifestyle the major cause of disease and illness, but we may be evolving ourselves into dysfunction, disease, and possibly out of existence. There is a better approach. We can take control of the evolutionary process and actually create ourselves to be healthier, to be better functioning, and to have the ability to sustain our species. We have the power in ourselves to create and sustain our health, to evolve in a positive manner.

Many of you, I am certain, know exactly what to do to reap the benefits of the adaptation toward health and fitness. For those of you who know what to do but are not practicing what they know, I want you to read this book and decide that it is time to refocus and regain your health. For those of you that are already healthy, fit, and self-sufficient, I want you to help me, because there are so many out there that are not experiencing health benefits now, or maybe never have. Please join me in inspiring those people to experience the feeling of a body that functions. Let everyone know that health comes from within, not from a practitioner that you may present yourself to. Let everyone know that it is within their power to be well.

For those of you who read this book, and who did not know or do not believe that there might be another way, please trust me long enough to complete an experiment. There is no gain without a challenge, but that challenge does not need to be overwhelming. Everyone will see benefits if they just take the first step and proceed to give it their best. Do not simply "try," since this gives you license to not to complete the task at hand. Remember the Nike slogan, "Just do it," and really experience how much you can benefit if you give your best shot. In my twenty years of practice, I have been surprised by so many people as I saw them discover that they could go beyond their current limits and beliefs. It continues to sadden me each time when people come into our clinic to be patients and explain to me all the symptoms and disease that they have grown accustomed to.

These patients have come to believe that living with symptoms and disease is their only choice. They actually begin to define themselves by the diseases, ICD codes, and symptoms that they are dealing with. As they discuss their history of diagnosed diseases, their list of medicine and supplements, and their years of suffering, I empathize and imagine how they must feel. "Doctor, I have this digestive problem, but the frequent headaches are normal, I am used to them. The joint pain I have all the time, I have dermatological creams for my skin problems, allergy medicine I take every day, something for my mood, and I also have something to control my blood pressure. Oh, and I have another pill to control my blood sugar. Will you help me with my digestion? I am taking antacids, but they do not work as well as they used to." Sometimes I have to hold back tears, and I want to tell this person that all these things are all related, and there is hope for correction instead of ongoing treatment.

These patients are not defined as a condition or disease; there is only evidence present of dysfunction in their biological systems. The human body never makes mistakes; it just responds in the best way that it can. Sometimes that response is not suitable for the person's current situation or their chosen lifestyle. Medications may be necessary in the short term and will ease their suffering, perhaps even save their lives; however, medications or even supplements are not necessarily correcting the situation or fixing the cause of their problem. In the case of a diabetic who does not produce insulin, or someone without a functioning thyroid, we may have to use medication for a lifetime. This is not the majority of cases, though. Patients are people first, and every person is experiencing a different interaction with the environment. Each person has their own paradigm that is different from everyone else's, as well as their individual and distinct stresses and responses.

In my opinion, "acceptance" of what is, is not an option. Therefore, each person requires an individualized strategy, which is based upon their own individual history. In functional medicine, we are taught to look for antecedents, triggering events, and perpetuators or mediators. The functional medicine model looks at the big picture and works to define the pattern of systems, mechanisms, and events that led up to the patient's current situation. This leads to a better strategy and a solution, since the source of the problem is better identified. There has never been a person born deficient in pharmaceutical medications; there is a bigger picture, taken in from higher up.

For more information on functional medicine, visit www.functionalmedicine.org.

If you have major complaints of symptoms and disease, please find a practitioner versed in this model to help you. I hope that this book outlines a new beginning for you. Please continue to follow with me as we explore the specifics on how to refine and implement your plan for wellness. It is about focusing on a lifestyle that is symbiotic with your body. You will be living in this vessel for your lifetime, and it will work properly if you allow it to. Health is a vital and positive thing that you create. It is living free of symptomology, free of medication, and even free of a multitude of nutritional supplements. Health, vitality, and wellness are gifts that you have the power to change.

When the patient discovers and perserveres with a good strategy, there is always then a point where this same patient looks me in the eye and states, "I have never in my life felt this good. Thank you." That is what I wish for you.

Additional Resources

For more information you can visit these websites:

www.functionalmedicine.org —The Institute For Functional Medicine
www.acam.org —American College for Advancement in Medicine
www.lifestylemedicine.org —American College of Lifestyle Medicine
www.worldhealth.net —American Academy of Anti-Aging Medicine
www.drhyman.com —Dr. Mark Hyman
www.mercola.com —Dr. Joseph Mercola
www.ewg.org —Environmental Working Group
www.austinwellnessclinic.com —Dr. Vincent Bellonzi

Thank you for reading this book. Please visit www.recklesshealth.com/book For a free bonus Audio CD, and more information on how to design your lifestyle. Please come and sign up for the newsletter and find resources for you new life.

Acknowledgments

I would like to thank all of the Functional Medicine practitioners who have guided me through the years, and been true companions to me on our path to understanding the patterns which are part of the biological systems which function together as life for the human being. Instead of the study of disease, we have designed a study of simultaneous systems, and are beginning to understand the mechanisms of life. This provides such advantages in helping people enjoy optimum vitality and wellness instead of ongoing treatments. Discerning the patterns is the only way that works to address the chronic diseases we all face. .

In particular I would like to thank Dr. Jeffrey Bland for his ability to see the patterns and guide us all to the right path. For many years he has foretold and taught a better way of truth.

I would like to thank Dr. Mark Hyman for being a driving force and educator who has inspired me as well.

I want to thank the compounding pharmacists and educators at Peoples Pharmacy and the Apothecary Shop in Austin for traveling with me on this path.

Thank You to the staff at the Austin Wellness Clinic for all they do to support me.

Thank you to Amanda Rooker, the editor of this book who helped my words create the message.

I would also like to thank my dear Sibylle, putting up with me, and encouraging me to write this book.

About the Author

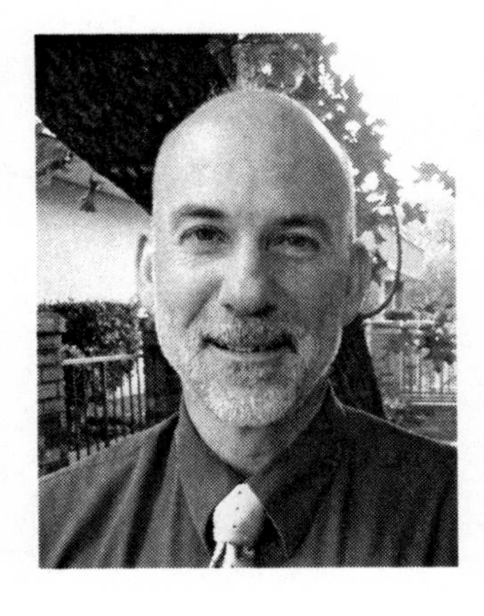

Dr. Vincent Bellonzi D.C., C.C.N., C.S.C.S, ACSM H/FI

An avid marathoner, Dr. Vincent Bellonzi developed an interest in optimal nutrition, health, and sports conditioning and as a result, he sought a Doctorate in Chiropractic and certifications as a personal trainer, cycling coach, running coach and nutritionist. He received his Doctorate from Los Angeles College of Chiropractic in 1991 and certified as a Health and Fitness instructor with the American College of Sports Medicine. He is also a certified Strength and Conditioning specialist and holds a B.S. in both Human biology and Nautical Industrial Technology.

Dr. Bellonzi is a Certified Clinical Nutritionist and has made the study of nutrition and exercise a central pillar of his practice and personal philosophy. He works with athletes at every level to provide sports conditioning and rehabilitation while treating conditions including headaches/migraines, fibromyalgia, chronic fatigue, neck and lower back injuries, shoulder, wrist, and knee injuries. Dr. Bellonzi provides human performance testing, nutritional counseling, personal training, coaching and metabolic testing services.

At the Austin Wellness Clinic, Dr. Bellonzi has specialized in nutrigenomics, or the interaction between genetics and nutrition. Along with Dr. Haest he has been developing protocols for adrenal function, anti-aging, hormone balance, human performance, allergy resolution, detoxification, and neurotransmitter balance.

CPSIA information can be obtained at www.ICGtesting.com
Printed in the USA
BVOW030355300413

319427BV00002B/28/P